ALL THINGS SLOTHS FOR KIDS

FILLED WITH PLENTY OF FACTS, PHOTOS, AND FUN TO LEARN ALL ABOUT SLOTHS

ANIMAL READS

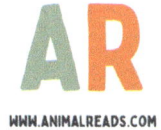

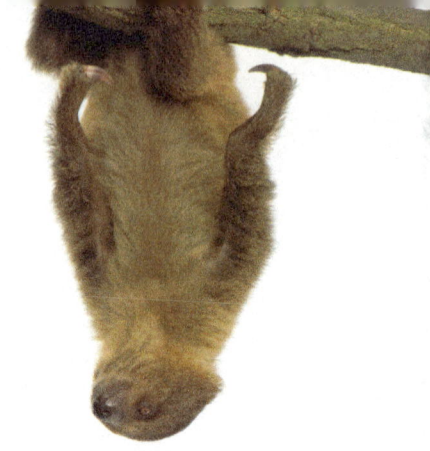

THIS BOOK BELONGS TO...

_____

_____

WWW.ANIMALREADS.COM

CONTENTS

Welcome to the Sloth House!	1
Different Types of Sloths	7
The History of Sloths	23
Where do Sloths live?	29
Characteristics and Appearance	33
Life Cycle	47
More Awesome Facts	57
Helping Sloths	61
Thank You!	67

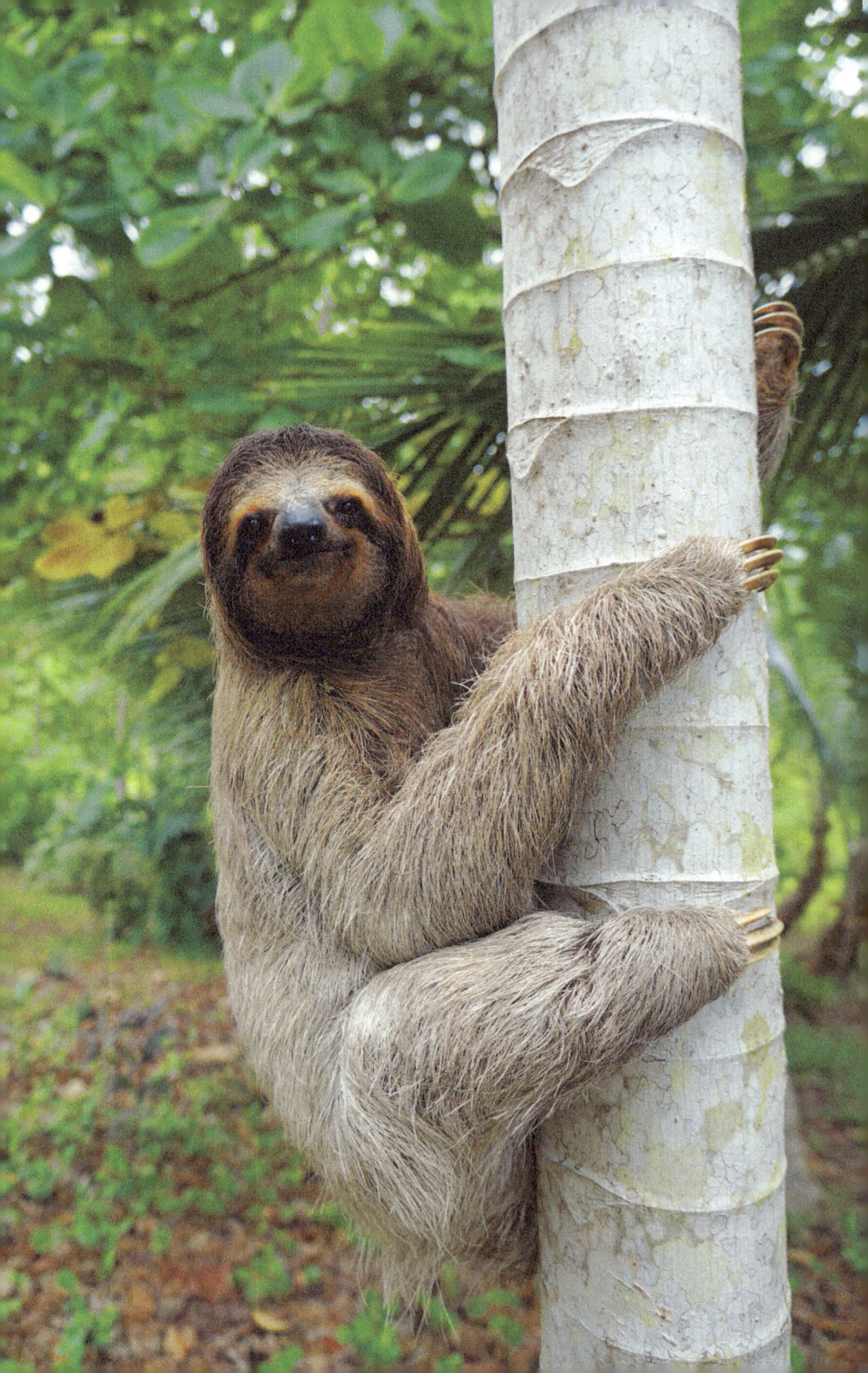

WELCOME TO THE SLOTH HOUSE!

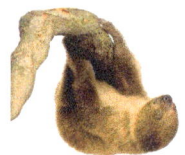

ave... you... ever... wondered... what... being... a... sloth... is... like?

WHEW! That was a slow sentence. *We wouldn't want to read a whole book written like that, would you?*

The first thing that probably comes to mind when you think about sloths is that they are slow. **Very, v e r y, slooooow**. Maybe hearing the word "*sloth*" also makes you think about people or animals who are lazy. Did you know the word "*sloth*" actually comes from a very old English word—*slouthe*—which means "laziness?"

But there is so much more to these delightful creatures than just their speed, *or more like... **lack of speed.*** Did you know sloths may hold the key to curing breast cancer? And sloths can hold their breath for 40 minutes underwater?

There are many, many things science still doesn't know about these cute, mysterious, and S-L-O-W mammals.

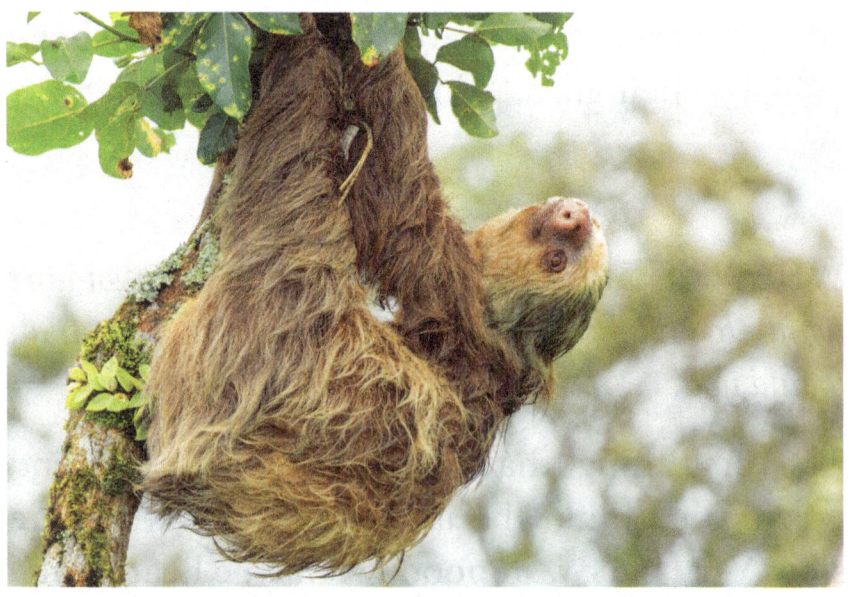

So, throw on some moss, hang from a tree, and come along for a wild, sloth-filled ride! *It might*

be a slow ride, but it will still be fun!

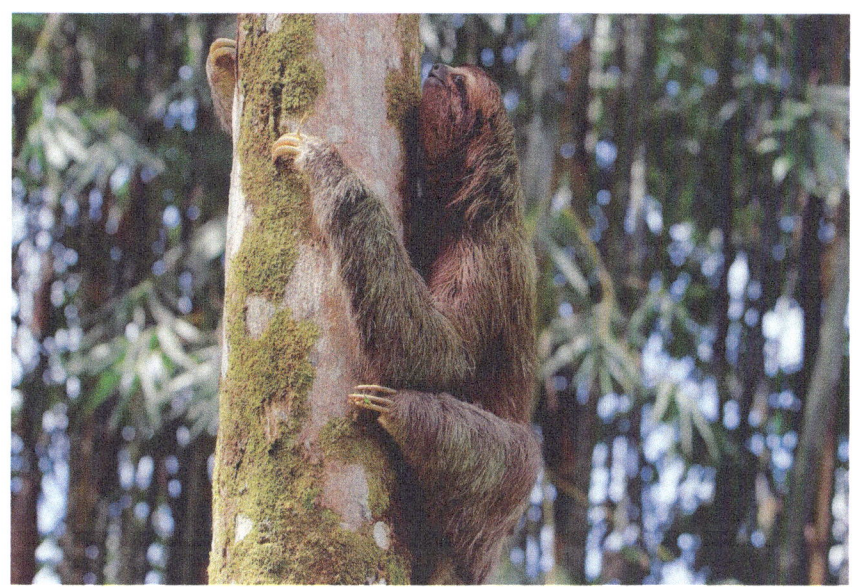

WHAT IS A SLOTH?

Sloths are mammals, which means they are warm-blooded animals with hair or fur, like humans. Sloths belong to the group of animals that are part of the arboreal neotropical xenarthran group. This group is also made up of anteaters and armadillos. All in all, there are 31 different species of anteaters, armadillos, and sloths that make up the living members of the xenarthran group.

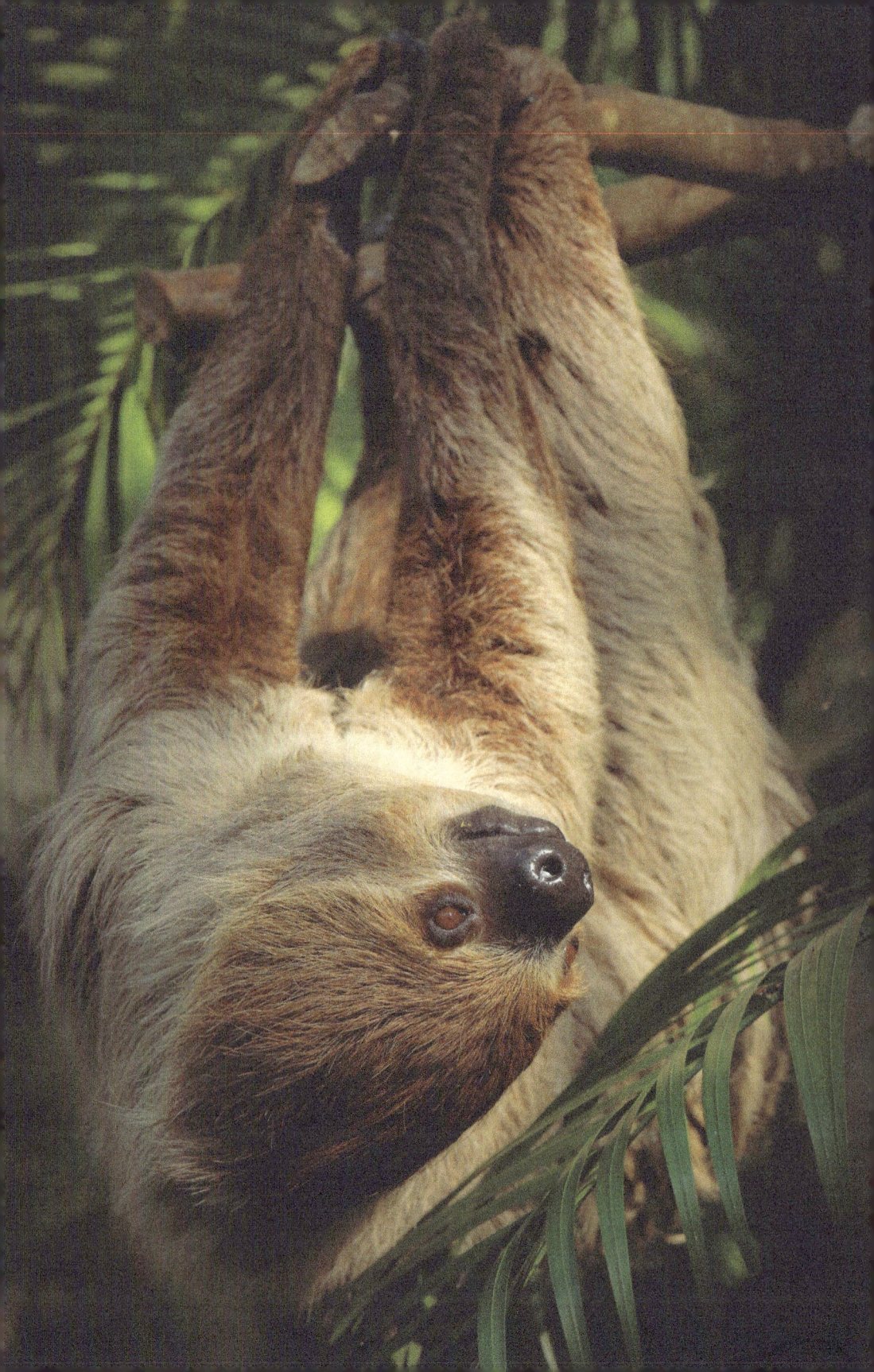

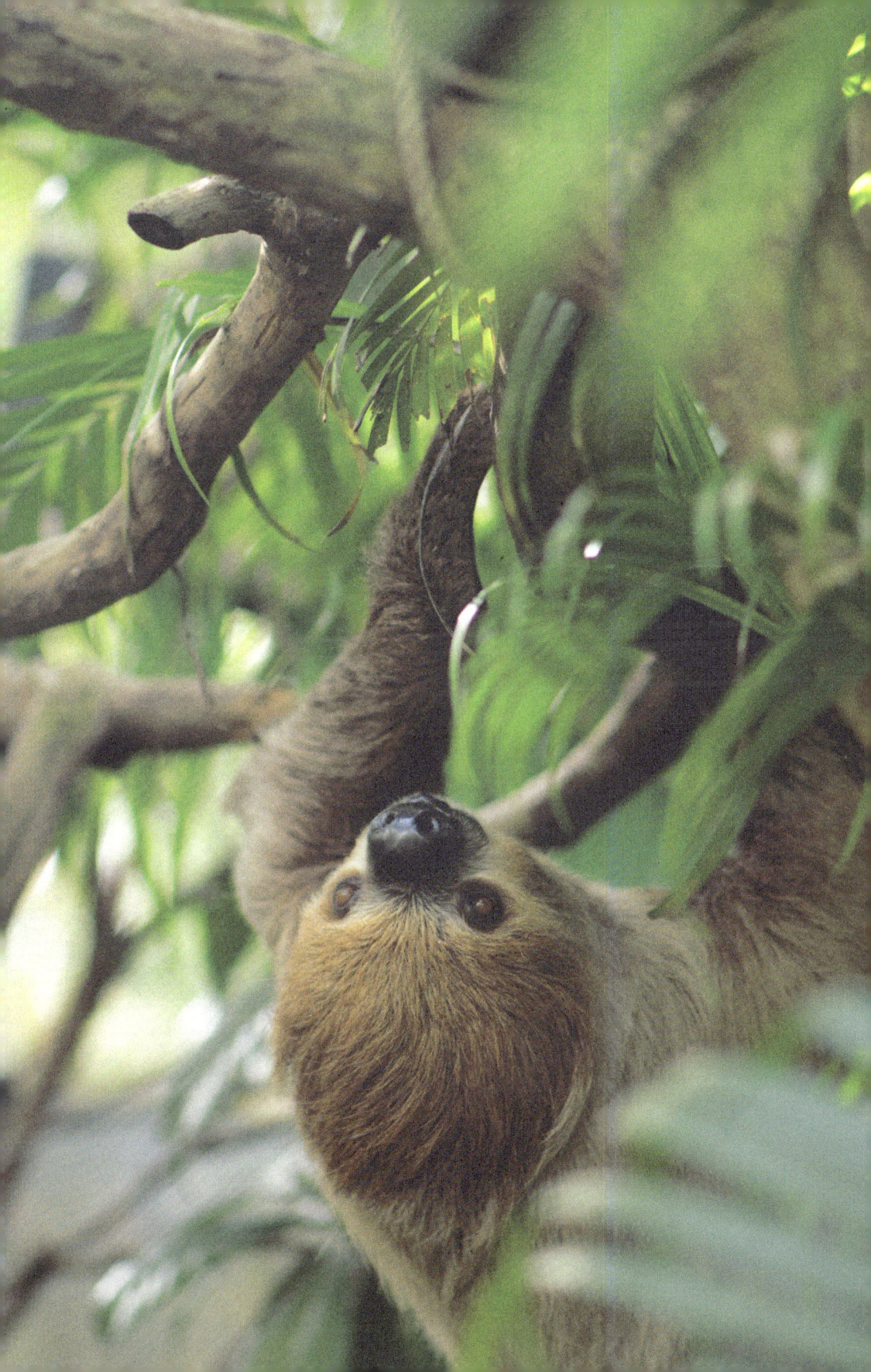

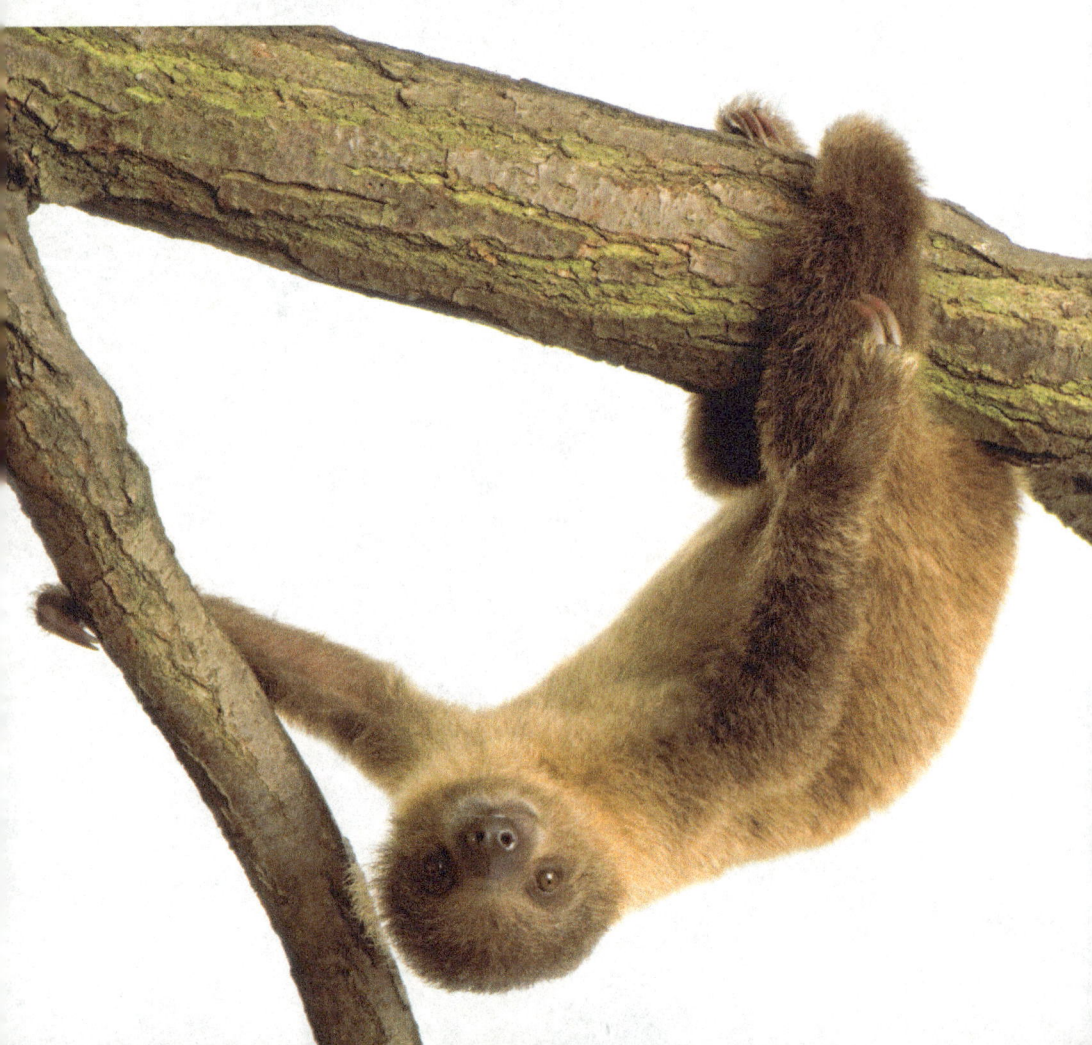

DIFFERENT TYPES OF SLOTHS
TWO-FINGERED AND THREE-FINGERED SLOTHS

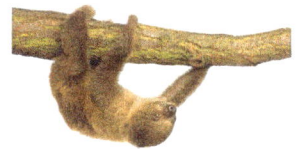

There are 6 living kinds of sloths in the world today. Sloths are broken up into two main groups, *"two-toed sloths"* and *"three-toed sloths."*

These groups are also called "two-fingered sloths" and "three-fingered sloths" because, actually, all sloths have three toes on their rear feet. But some have two toes/fingers on their front feet, and some have three/toes fingers on their front feet.

Having one less finger may not seem like a big difference, but there are actually quite a few differences between these two groups. Scientists now know that these two groups of sloths actually evolved from different prehistoric ancestors entirely. Because of this, two-fingered and three-fingered sloths are only very distantly-related. Maybe like you and your fourth cousin. Only with these sloths they are even less connected!

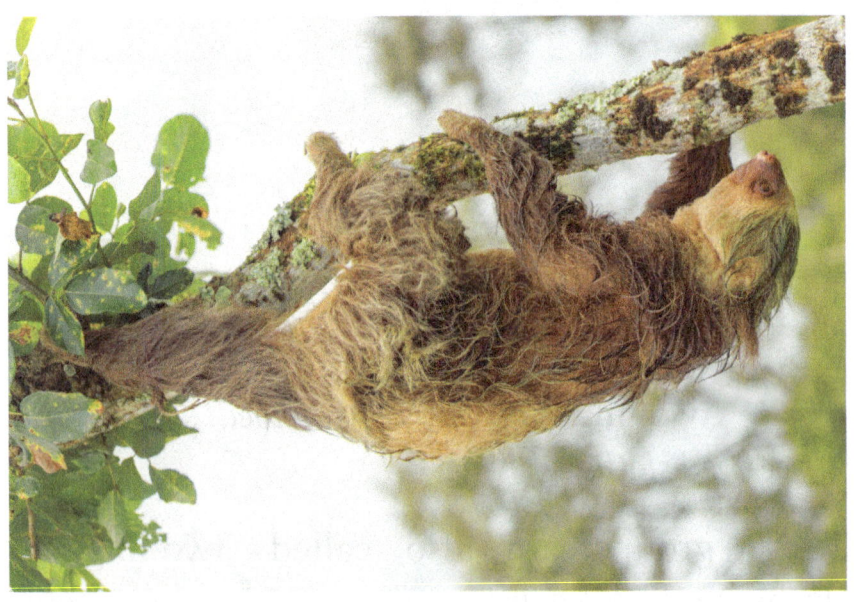

The fact that both groups of sloths look and act similar to each other is because of something called "*convergent evolution.*" This is when two separate species both adapt or change similarly because they live in the same ecosystem.

So, two different kinds of prehistoric sloths evolved in many of the same ways, and now we have these two modern groups of sloths—two-fingered sloths and three-fingered sloths.

Let's take a quick look at these lovable slow-pokes and get an overview of the two main groups of sloths and the 6 species of sloths that are around today:

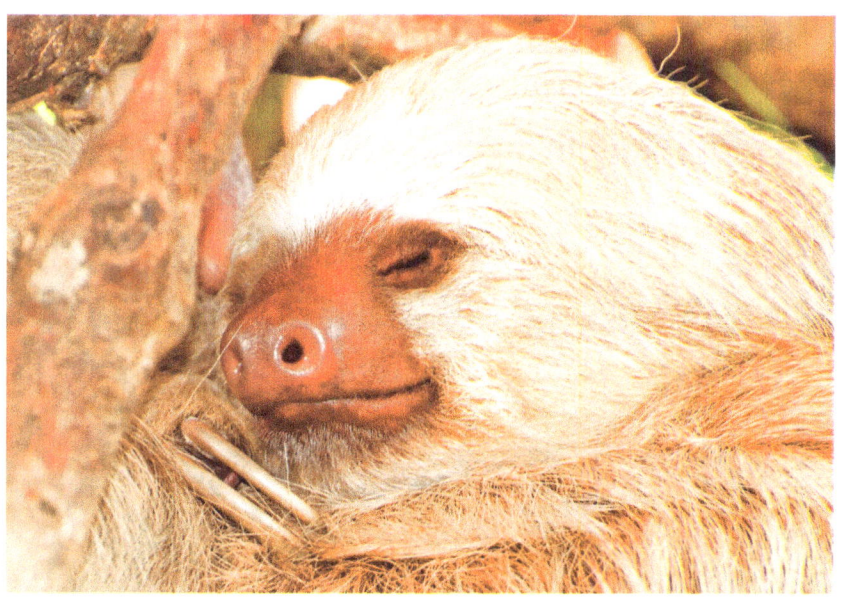

TWO-FINGERED SLOTHS

- They have long hair, which can come in different colors depending on where they live
- They have a longer nose that almost looks pig-like
- They are more active and can move faster than three-fingered sloths
- They are much larger
- There are only 2 species of two-fingered sloths still living today

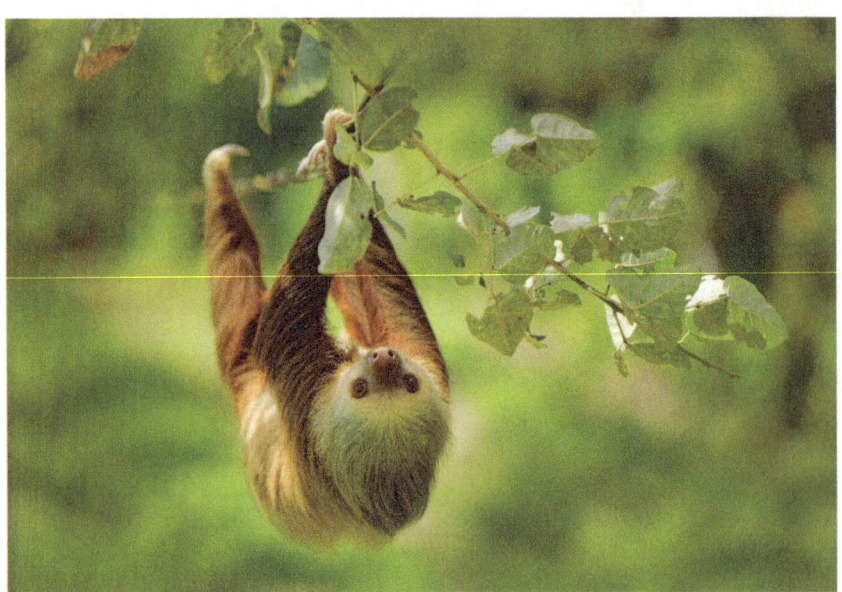

HOFFMANN'S SLOTH *(CHOLOEPUS HOFFMANNI)*

These sloths can be found from Honduras down to northern Bolivia. Hoffmann's sloth usually comes in a color that is a mixture of light brown, tan, and blonde. The hair on this species is often longer, and like all kinds of sloths, their hair parts down the middle of their stomach. This is especially handy as it allows rainwater to run down the hair and not pool on the sloth's stomach as it hangs upside down. They have round heads and relatively flat faces. Hoffmann's sloth are not currently endangered.

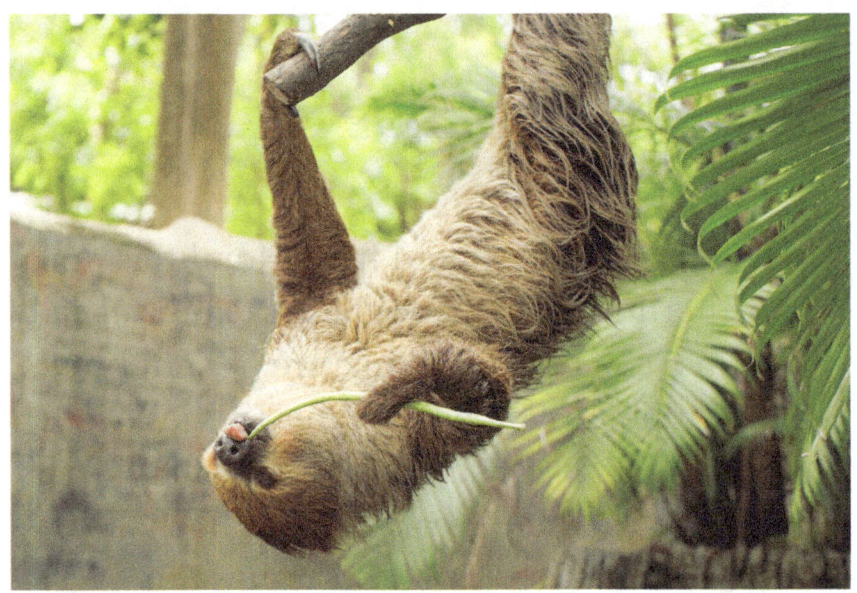
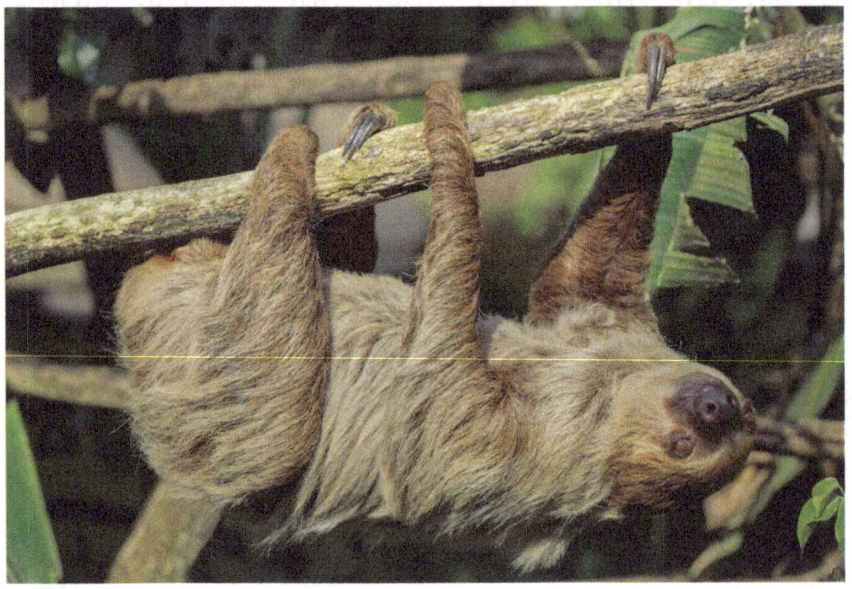

LINNAEUS'S SLOTH *(CHOLOEPUS DIDACTYLUS)*

These sloths look a lot like Hoffmann's sloth, but they are darker colored on their hands, feet, and nose. This species of sloth is the most common to find in zoos. If you've ever seen a sloth in real life, it was probably an example of Linnaeus's sloth. Thankfully, these sloths are also not endangered.

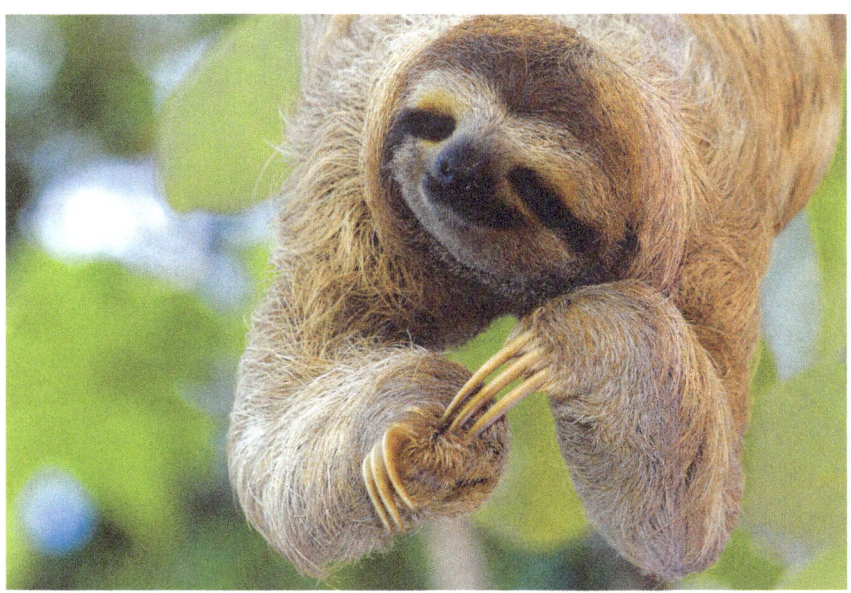

THREE-FINGERED SLOTHS

- These sloths have little heads and always look like they're smiling
- All but 1 of these species have a dark marking (*or mask*) around their eyes
- They have very long arms compared to their legs. Their legs are only half as long as their arms
- With their extra neck bones (*vertebra*), they can turn their heads 270 degrees
- There are 4 living species of three-fingered sloths around today

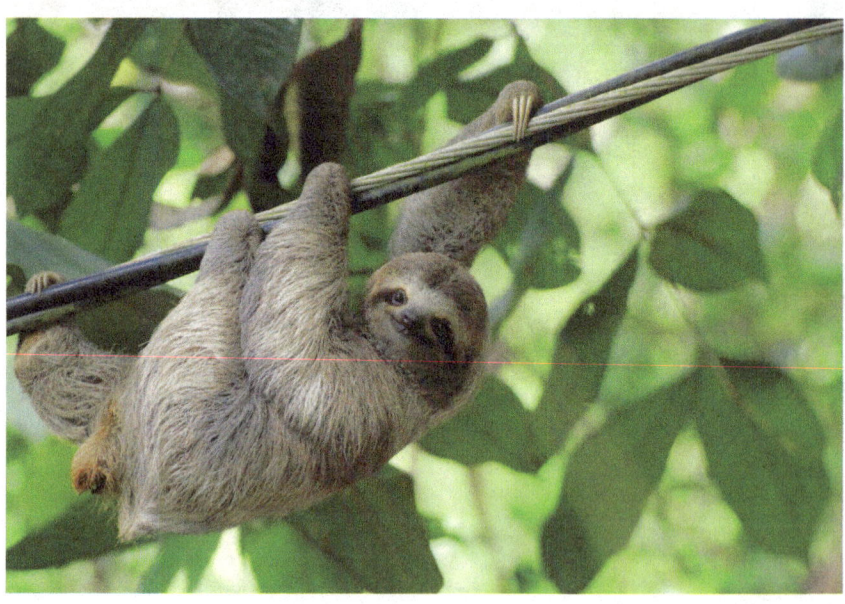

BROWN-THROATED SLOTH (*BRADYPUS VARIEGATUS*)

The brown-throated sloth is found throughout the northern half of South America, from Costa Rica all the way down through Brazil. They have a white forehead and usually have brown or gray and white fur. This species is around the same size as an average cat. Fortunately, these commonly found sloths are not endangered and have a conservation status of "least concern."

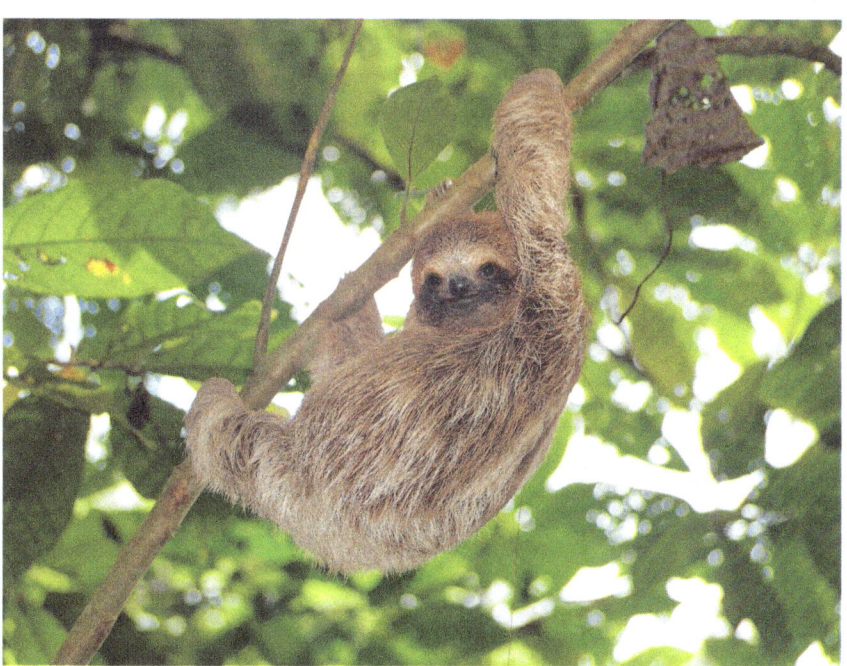

PYGMY SLOTH (*BRADYPUS PYGMAEUS*)

These sloths are the most endangered of all the sloth species and one of the most critically endangered mammals currently in the world. Almost half the size of the brown-throated sloth, they look very similar to this species except for their tiny size. The pygmy sloth was only found to be its own species in 2001 and are only found on a very small island in Panama.

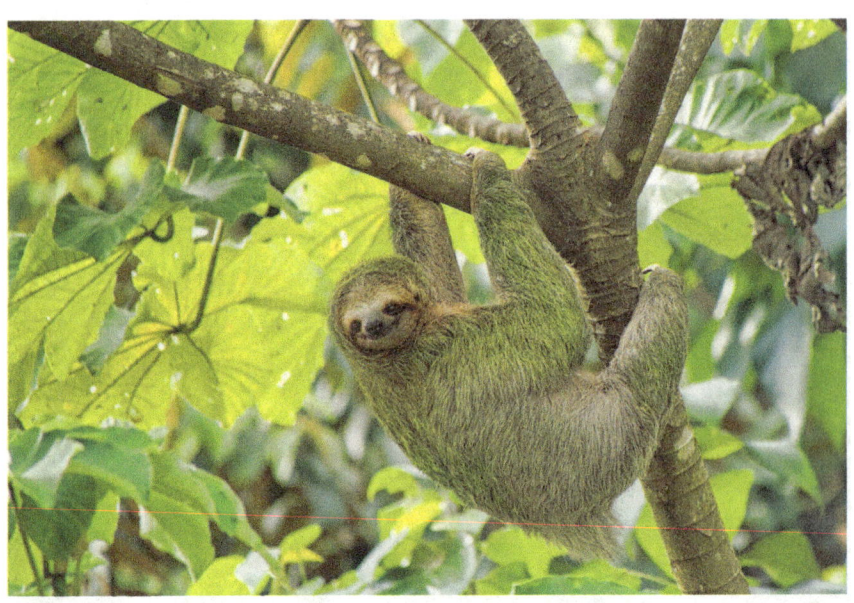

PALE-THROATED SLOTH (*BRADYPUS TRIDACTYLUS*)

The pale-throated sloth looks very similar to the brown-throated sloth, except for the pale yellow section on its throat. The adults develop black-tinged gray fur with darker areas on their backs. This sloth species lives in the northern area of South America, in the countries of Colombia and the western half of Venezuela. Thankfully, this sloth species is also not endangered at this time.

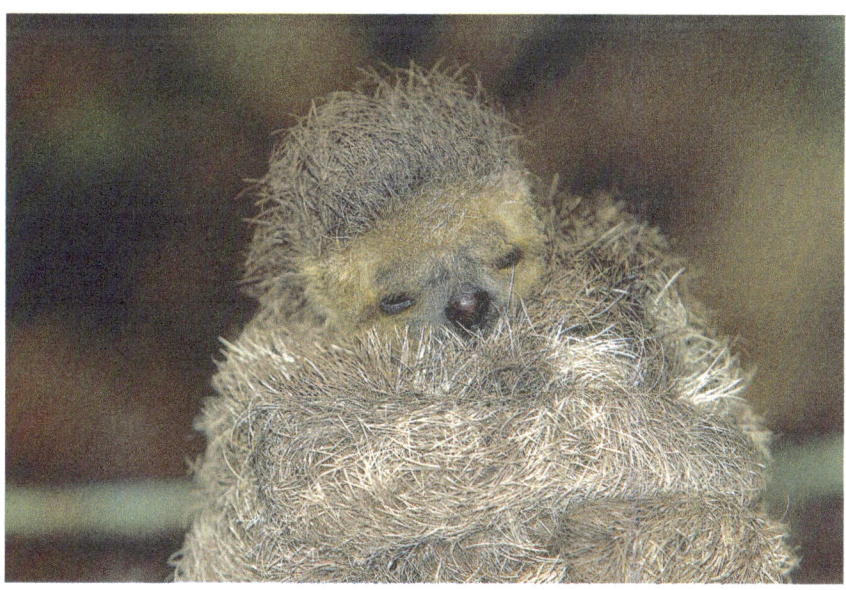

MANED SLOTH (*BRADYPUS TORQUATUS*)

This species of sloth is currently considered vulnerable in their conservation status. The only known habitat for the maned sloth is the coastal forests of Brazil that border the Atlantic Ocean. They are vulnerable because of loss of habitat. They have a "mane" of black hair around their neck, and they are the only three-fingered sloth not to have the dark mask markings around their eyes. These sloths are often dark brown or gray, and they are also the biggest of all three-fingered sloths.

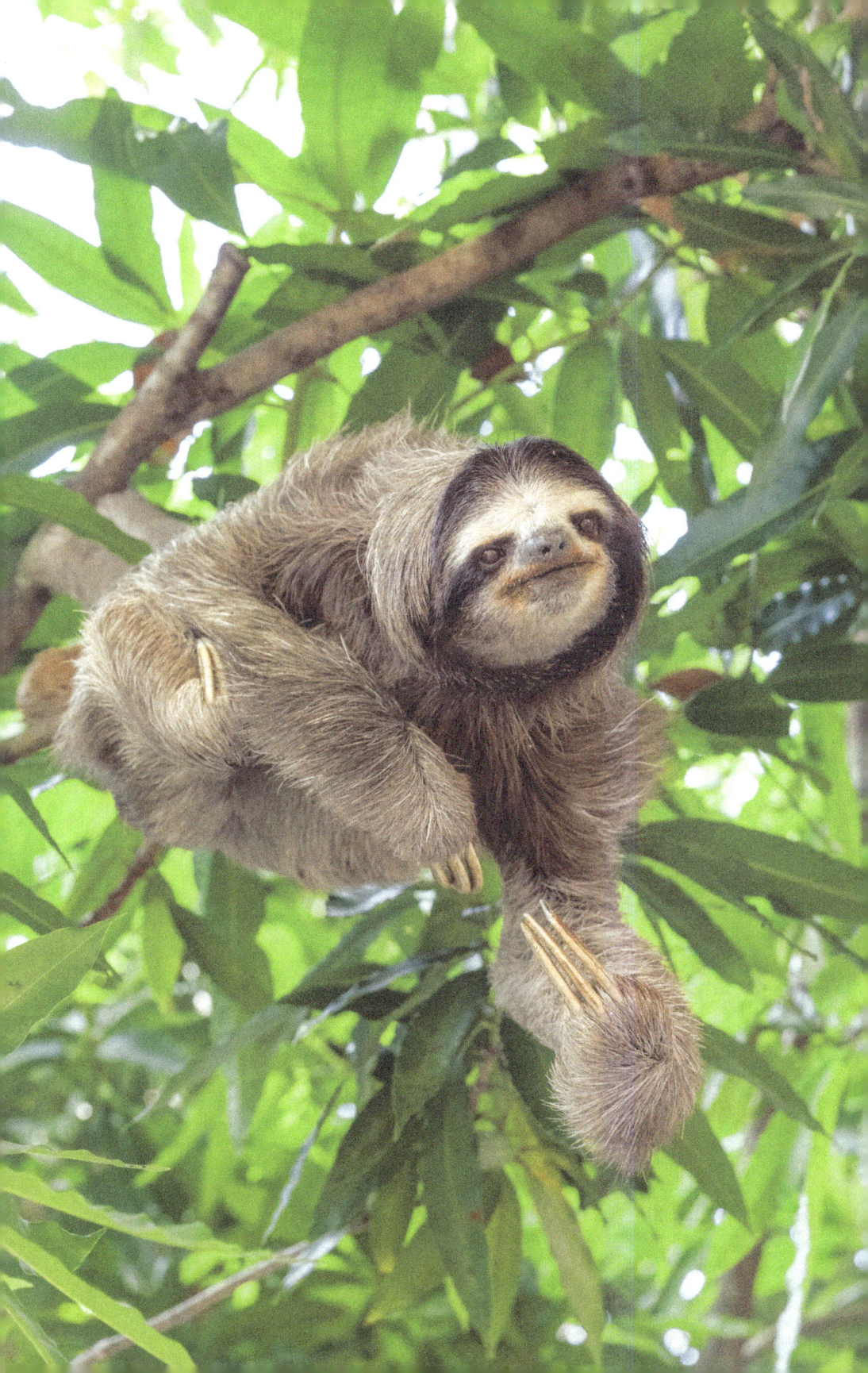

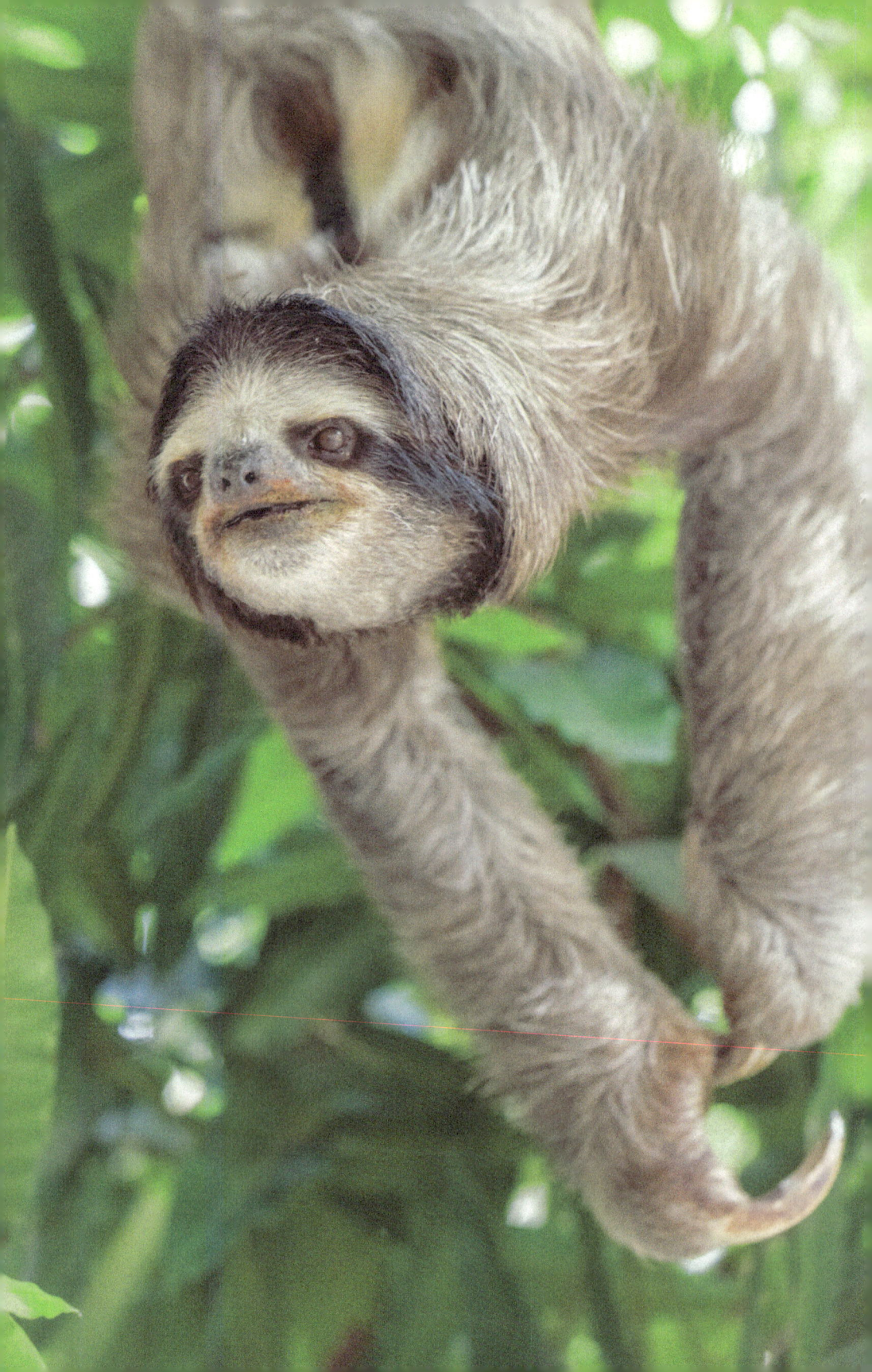

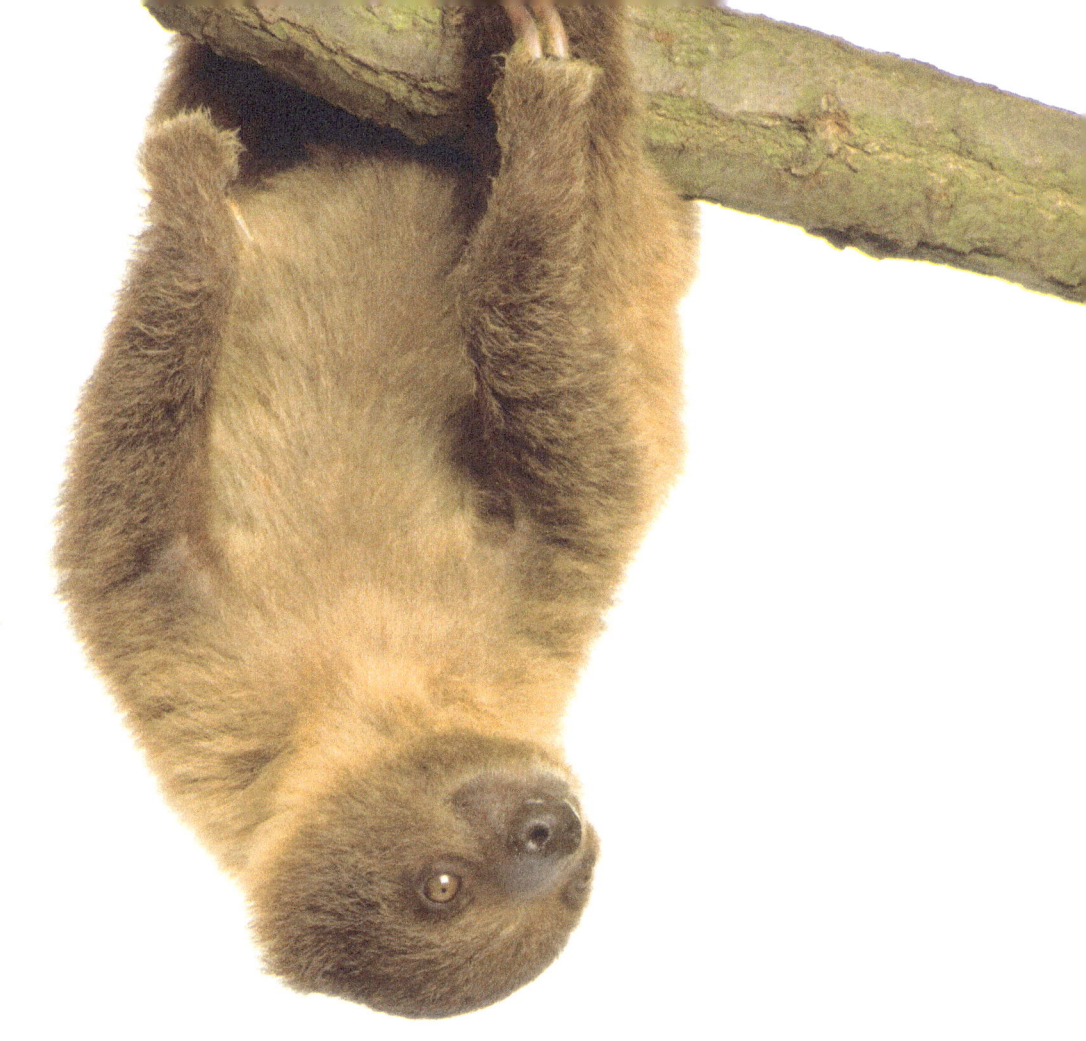

THE HISTORY OF SLOTHS

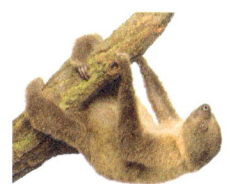

Sloths have been around for millions of years. There were many different species of prehistoric sloths that once lived all the way up to North America. The earliest sloths were all ground-dwellers and all of today's modern sloths evolved from these giant ground sloths.

One of the most impressive early sloths was the *Megatherium*. These sloths were ground-dwellers and the size of elephants! The translation of the Greek word for these huge sloths means *"great beast."* The Megatherium lived in the grasslands of modern southern Bolivia. These huge sloths, also known as the giant ground sloths, could grow to be 12 feet tall and 20 feet long, and they could weigh as much as 5,000 pounds.

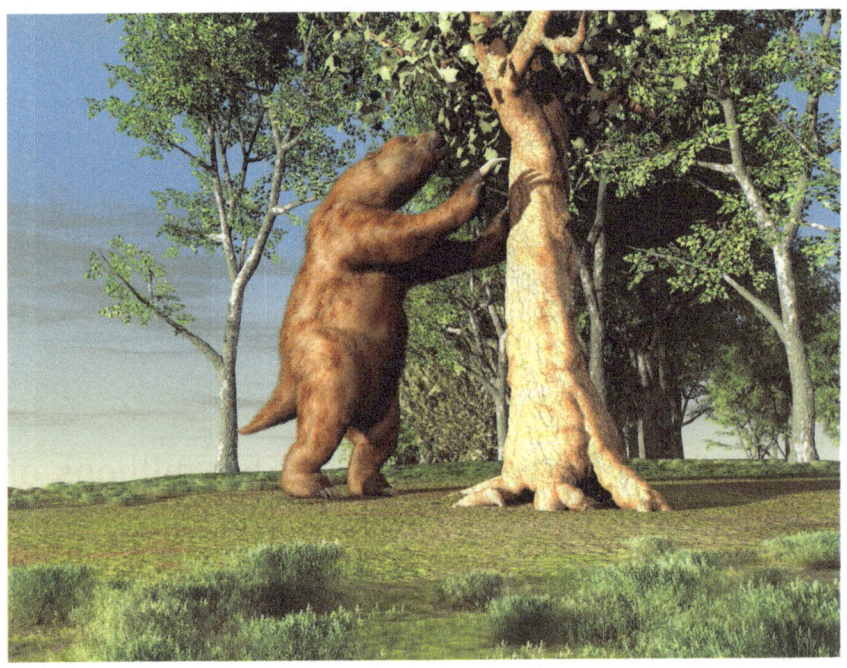

Unfortunately, humans from long ago may be to blame for why these large, ground-dwelling sloths and similar species went extinct. There is evidence that ground sloths were hunted and used for food. Their disappearance in both North and South America seems to line up with the arrival of humans to those areas around 11,000 years ago. The Megatherium first showed up around the early Pliocene period and lasted through the end of the Pleistocene period, which is also called the Ice Age.

Some species of these ancient ground sloths were even *semi-aquatic*, which means they lived part of their time in the water. These water-dwelling sloths were good swimmers and fed on seagrasses that grew on the ocean floor.

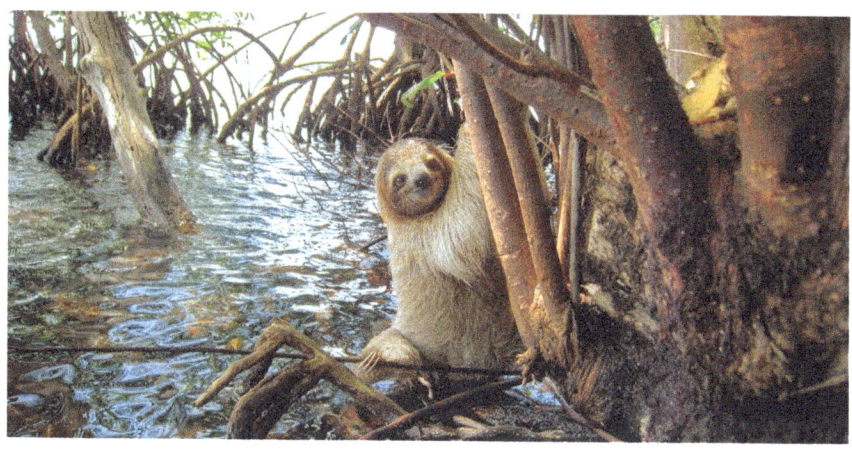

One now extinct species, the *Thalassocnus sloth*, first showed up around 8 million years ago. This swimming sloth had long claws that it probably used to claw its way along the ocean floor with as it looked for food. This species of sloth went extinct around 4 million years ago. But it seems that modern sloths did keep something from their water-loving ancestors.

Modern sloths still enjoy the water and are also good swimmers. Because the sloths have so much gas in their large stomachs, they can float really well. Amazingly, sloths can swim three times faster than they can move on land (or in trees). And because sloths have such long necks, they can easily keep their heads above the water. Swimming is a necessary part of life for a sloth. Because the rainforests are often filled with lakes and rivers, sloths need to cross these water barriers to get to new territory. Sloths can't jump from tree to tree the way monkeys do, so they must swim.

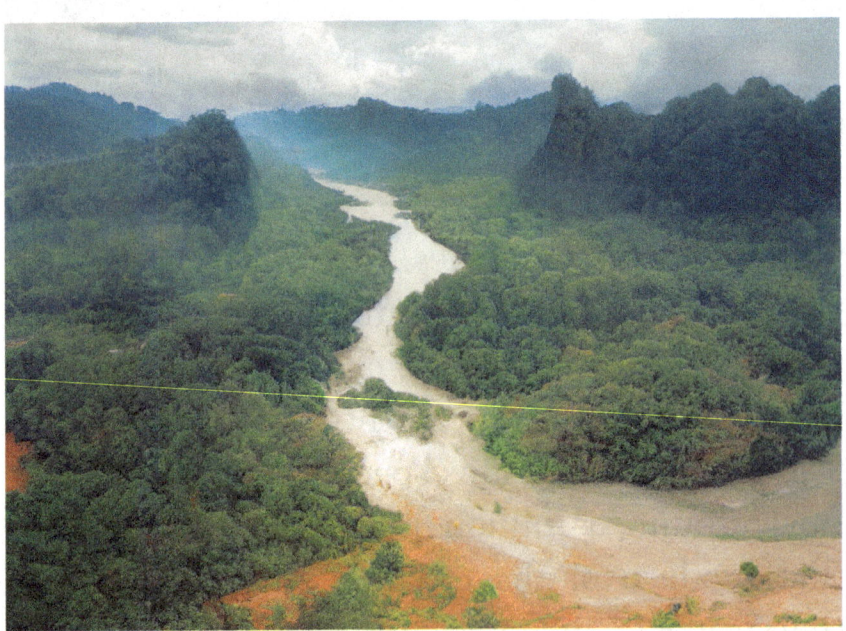

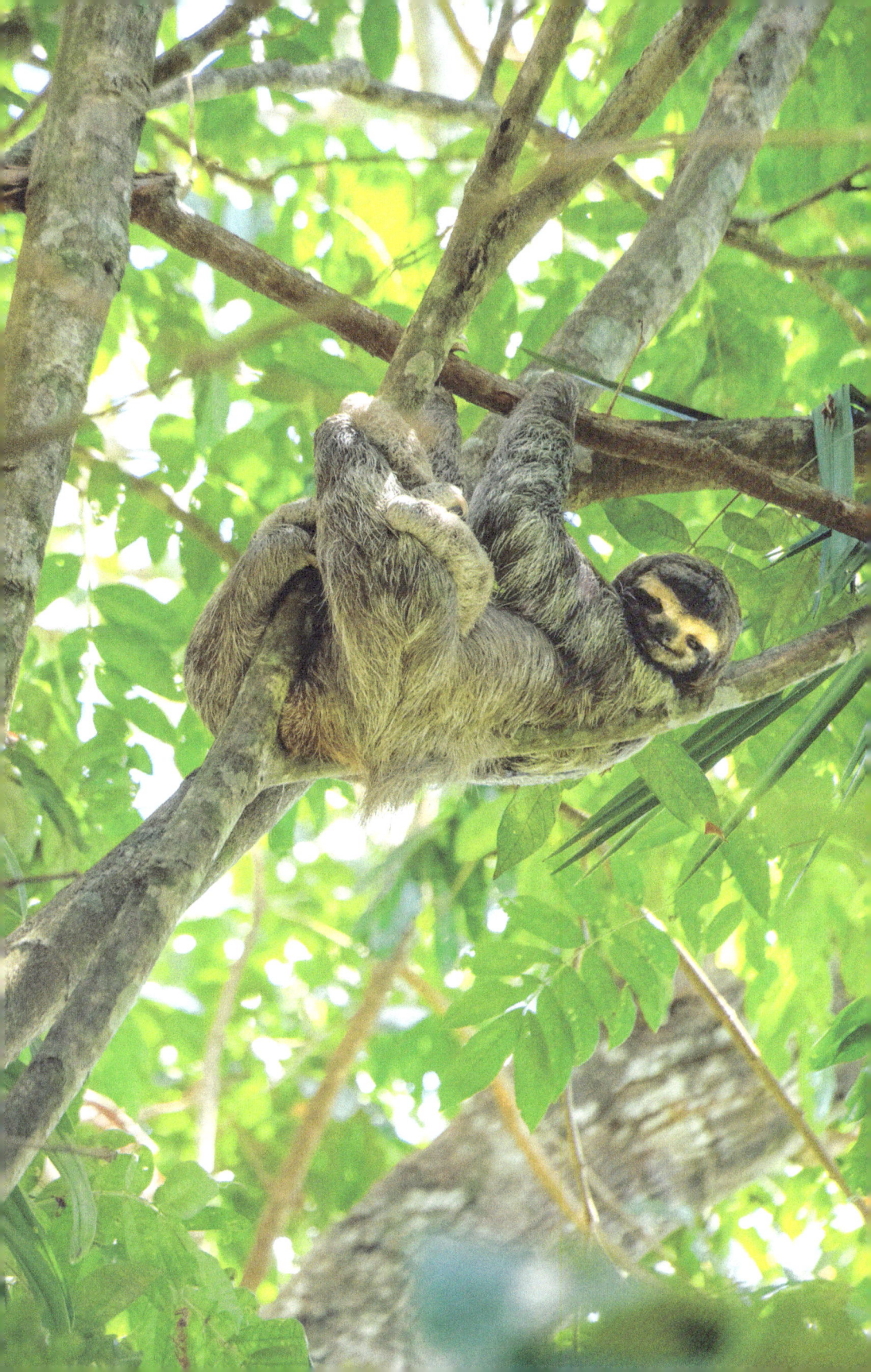

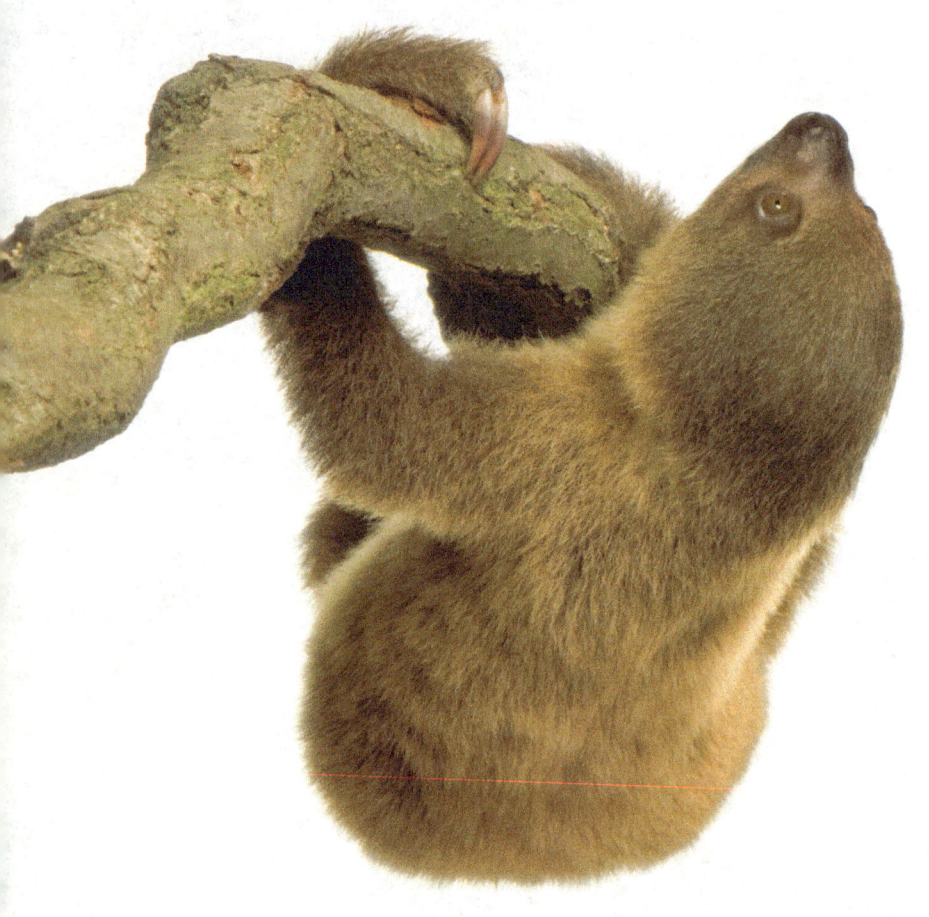

WELCOME TO THE SLOTH SIDE...

We nap here!

WHERE DO SLOTHS LIVE?

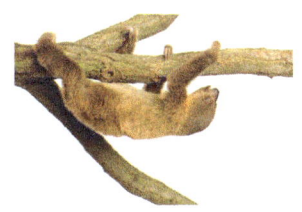

Ever wonder why you've never seen a sloth hanging from a tree in your town? There's a good reason for that. Sloths need a very special habitat to survive. The tropical rainforests of Central and South America are the only place we find sloths.

Although sloths don't live in many places, where they do live, they seem to thrive. The Barro Colorado Island in the country of Panama has an incredible number of sloths. In fact, out of all the arboreal mammals on the island (*that means out of all the mammals that live in trees*), sloths make up 70% of these animals.

If you dangle over the side of your bed or couch and look at the ceiling, you will get a look at the world through the eyes of a sloth. **That's right!** Sloths spend most of their time hanging upside down from tree limbs high in the forest.

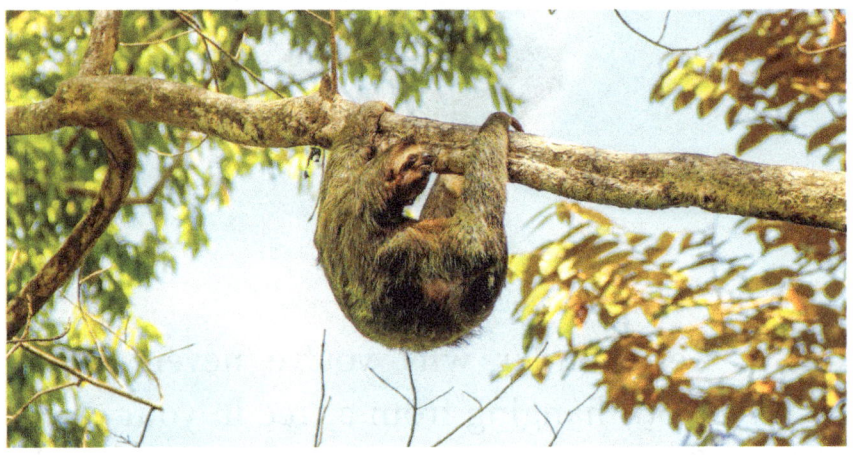

Even though they are mammals, sloths rely on a warm environment to help get the heat they need, which is another reason they live in tropical rainforests. Sloths are a rare kind of mammal that is heterothermic, which means their body temperature may change drastically based on the environmental temperature. A sloth's body temperature can be as low as 68 degrees Fahrenheit and as high as 95 degrees Fahrenheit.

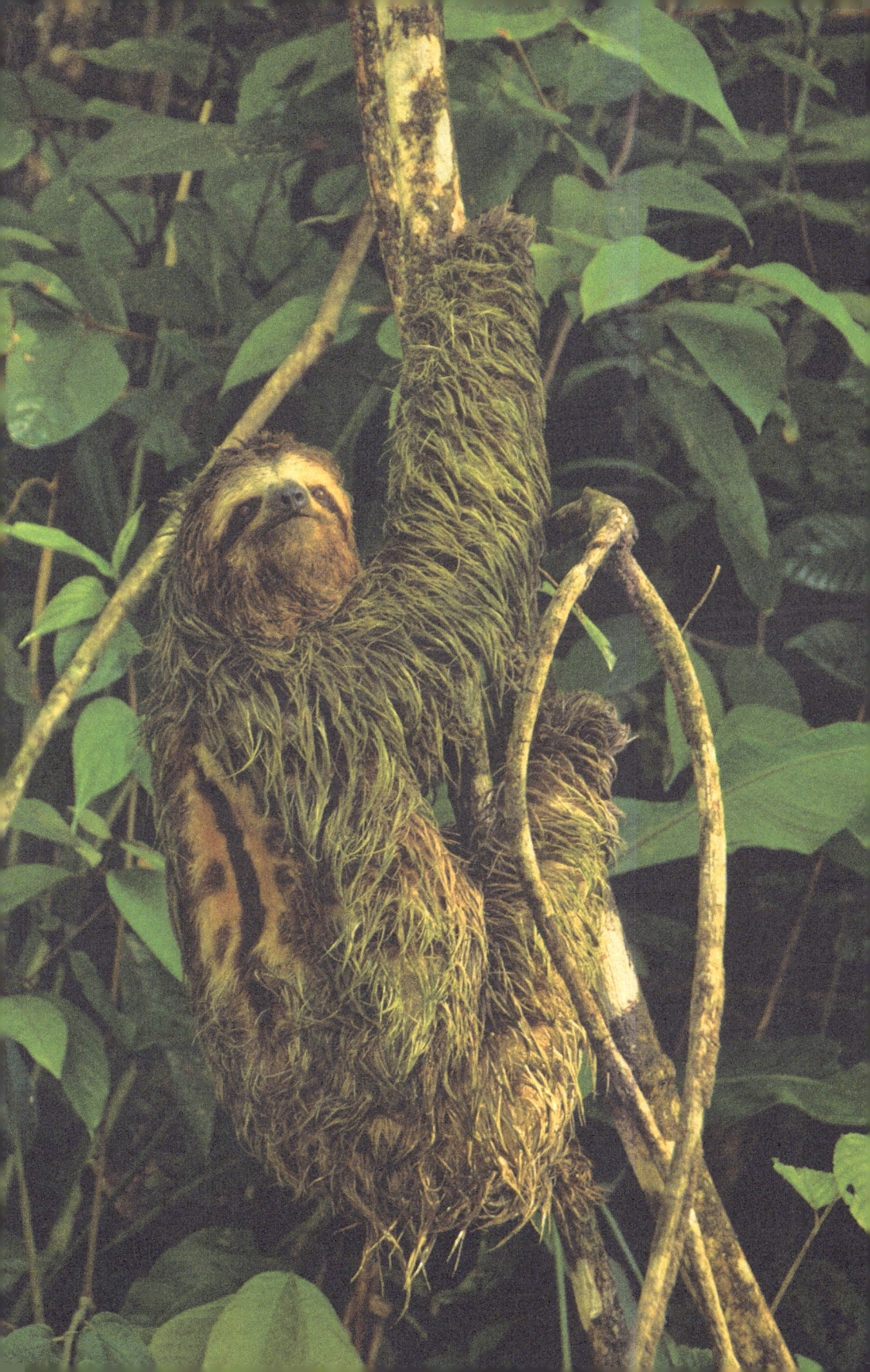

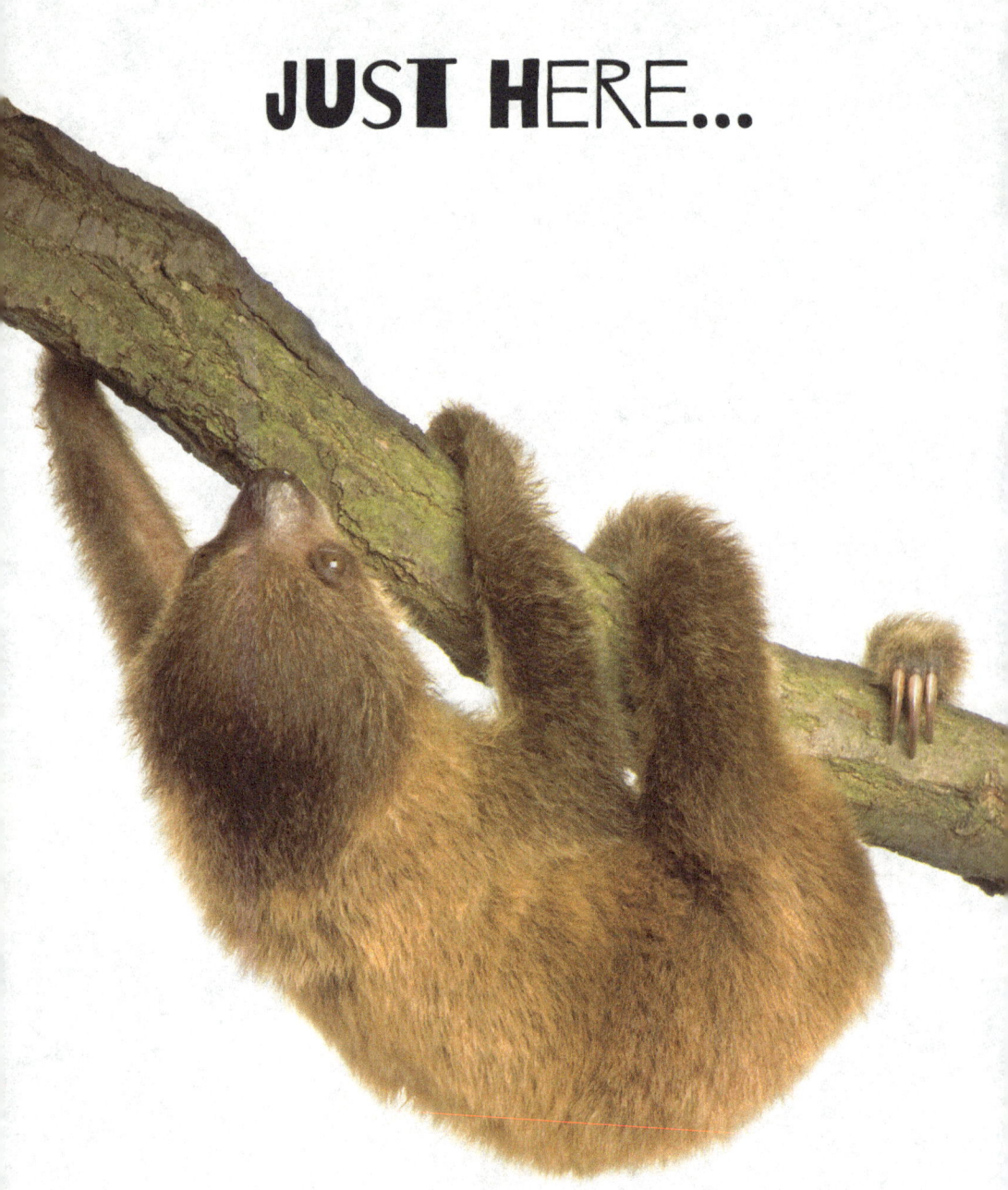

CHARACTERISTICS AND APPEARANCE

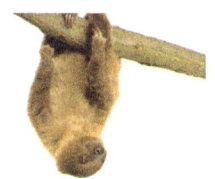

There are few animals cuter than the smiling sloth. Sloths are covered in fur, have small heads, big noses, and look like they're smiling. All sloths have three toes on their back feet and either two or three toes on their front feet. They have very long arms, which are perfect for hanging from trees.

Sloths aren't as big as you might think. Most sloths are around 24 to 31 inches long, and they only weigh from 7 to 17 lbs. *That is probably only the size and weight of your school backpack!* Imagine what fun it would be if you walked into your class with a sloth on your back instead.

If you did take a sloth to school, it would probably need glasses. Sloths can't see very well, although they can see in color. Especially in bright sunlight, a sloth is almost blind.

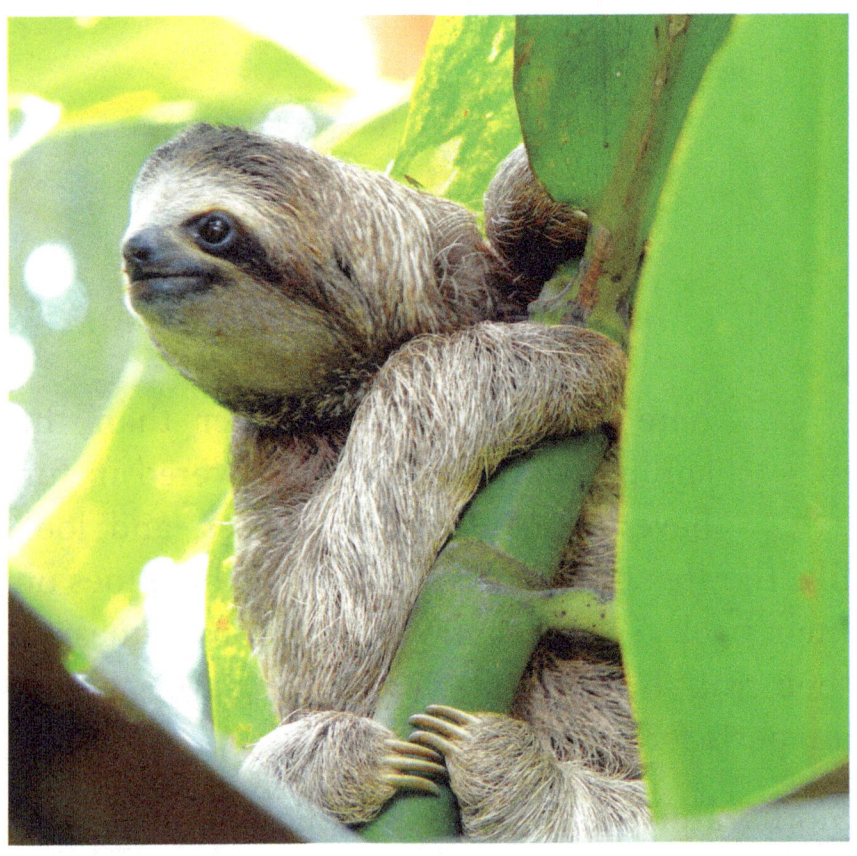

You would also need to sit very close to the teacher because sloths can't hear well either. But even though they can't see or hear well at all, they can smell and feel. This is how a sloth finds food, and it also uses its sense of smell to know when a predator is nearby.

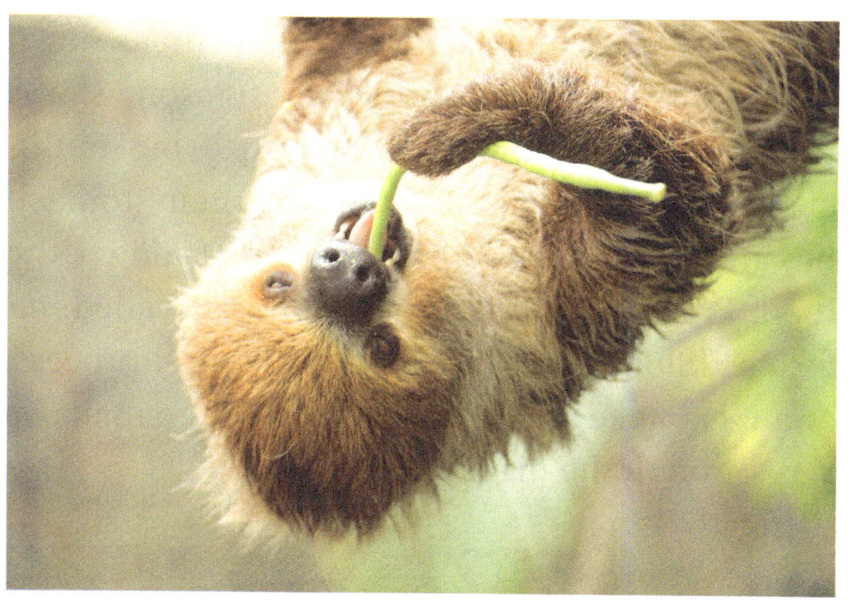

DIET AND METABOLISM

Sloths have a super-slow metabolism. *What does that mean?* It means sloths are very slow at converting the energy from food into energy their body uses. Because they are so slow, sloths don't have to eat as much as a mammal with a high metabolism, like a goat. However, because of their slow metabolism, sloths do not have very much energy, and they don't move very fast.

Three-fingered sloths only eat leaves, which is another reason they have evolved to have a slower metabolism. Leaves don't give as much energy as other foods, and they don't break down very easily once eaten. For this reason, sloths process their food very slowly in a big multi-chambered stomach. This means their stomach has different "*rooms*" that help break down the food. Processing food in your body is called "*digestion*." Sloths have a very slow digestive process, and it can take a month for their food to make its way through the digestive tract.

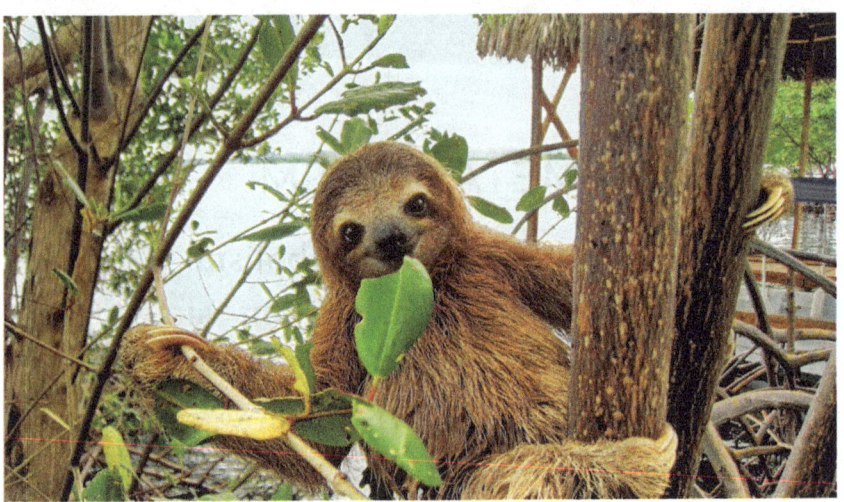

Three-fingered sloths usually eat from one main tree and then climb down once a week to poop near the base of that tree. There are all kinds of theories as to why sloths decide to take the risky move of coming down from the safety of their tree just to use the bathroom.

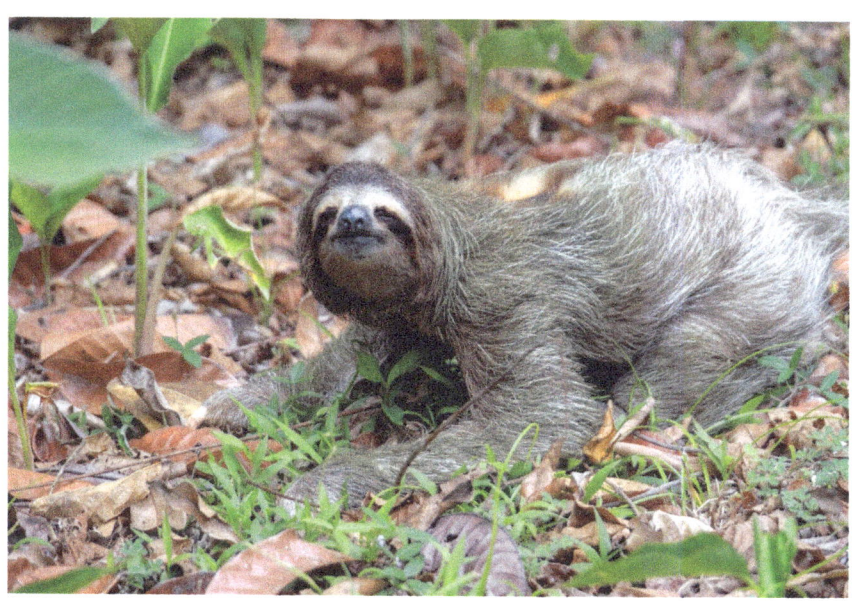

Some scientists wonder if this is a way the sloth helps to fertilize its tree and keep it healthy by pooping at the base of the tree and burying it. Other theories are that sloths poop on the ground because that's what their ground-dwelling ancestors did. Or perhaps sloths prefer to drop their droppings on the ground to spread scents and attract mates.

Two-fingered sloths have a much more varied diet than their three-fingered relatives. They eat leaves as well, but also add in fruits, insects, and even lizards! These sloths will also eat *carrion*, which is other dead animals they come across. They are *omnivores*, which means they eat both plants and meat.

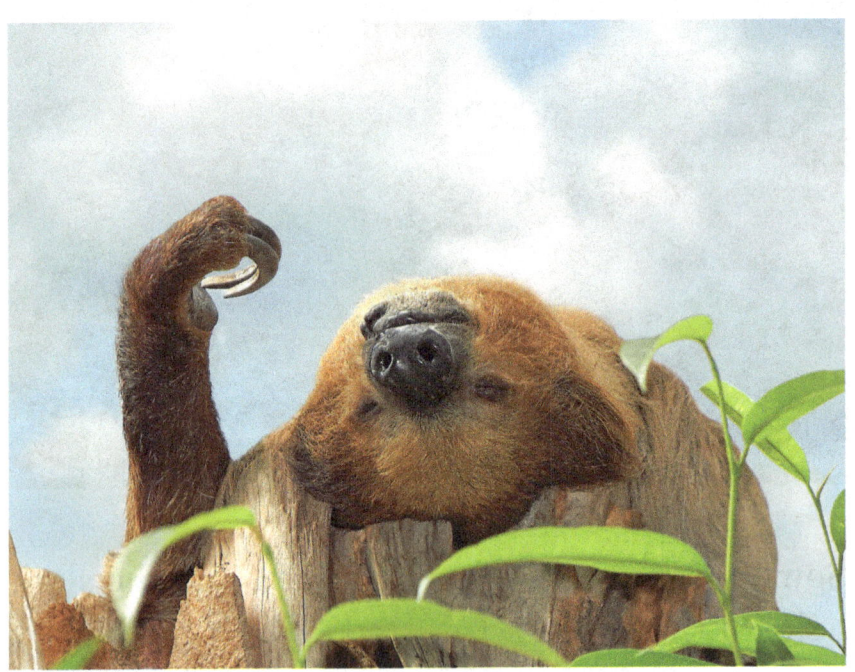

STAYING ALIVE AS A SLOTH

Because sloths move so little, plants actually grow on their fur, such as green algae. But the sloths don't mind. The algae, which also grows on trees, acts as a perfect camouflage for these tree-dwelling friends so they can blend into their green rainforest habitat.

Blending in is important if you're a sloth. As you've probably already figured out, sloths aren't very good at out-running predators who want to eat them. They also aren't cut out for fighting back.

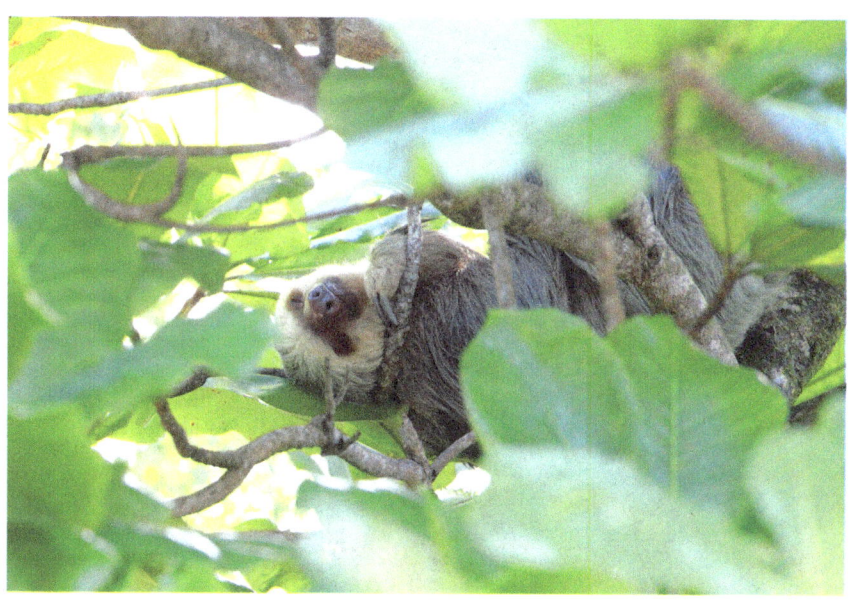

So, what's their best defense? **You guessed it...** *hiding!* This is where moving slowly comes in handy. An animal that is not moving or moving very slowly is very hard to see, especially for predators who typically rely on fast movement to see their prey.

But who would want to hurt a sloth? For starters, tree-climbing wild cats like jaguars and ocelots would love nothing more than to find a tasty sloth dinner. Then there are also threats from the sky, such as the harpy eagle.

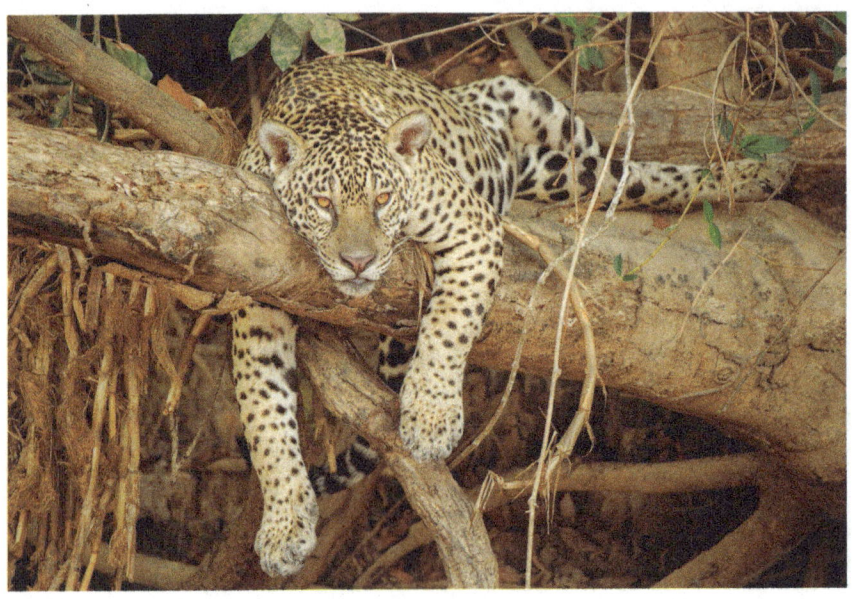

But three-fingered sloths have evolved another cool trick besides camouflage to avoid predators. Because they have an extra few vertebra in their neck (*extra bones that most other mammals don't have*), sloths can turn their head an impressive

270 degrees. This means a sloth can turn its head and smell approaching danger much better than most animals can. While they can't turn all the way around like an owl can (360 degrees), this is still an impressive range! As a comparison, you can only turn your head 90 degrees from side to side.

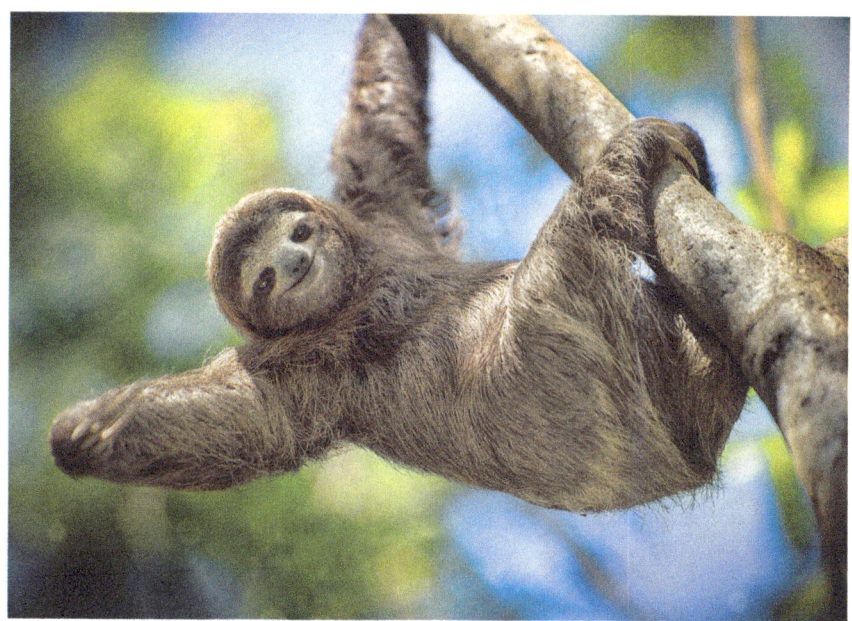

JUST HANGING AROUND!

As you already learned, sloths spend much of their time hanging upside down high in trees. This is where sloths spend their whole lives! Eating, sleeping, mating, and giving birth are just some of the activities sloths do upside down.

Have you ever hung upside down from the monkey bars on a playground? We bet your hands got pretty tired after just a little while! *So, how do sloths do it?* How do they hang from trees for hours on end without any breaks and not get tired?

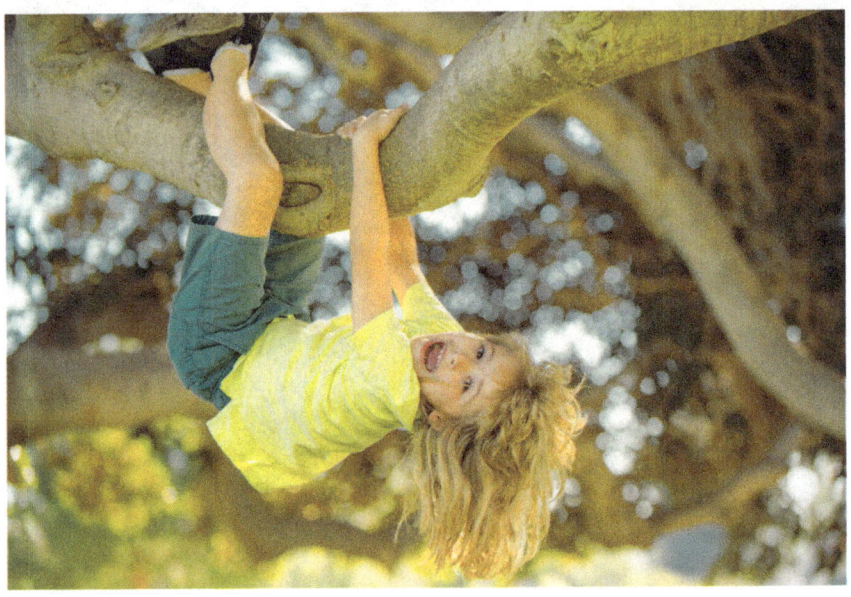

Sloths have developed a very special way to hang in trees without using too much energy. For instance, the *tendons* in their hands can lock in place. Tendons are a kind of muscle. When you combine these locking tendons with the long and rounded claw-like nails the sloth has, they can hang out all day long without getting tired at all.

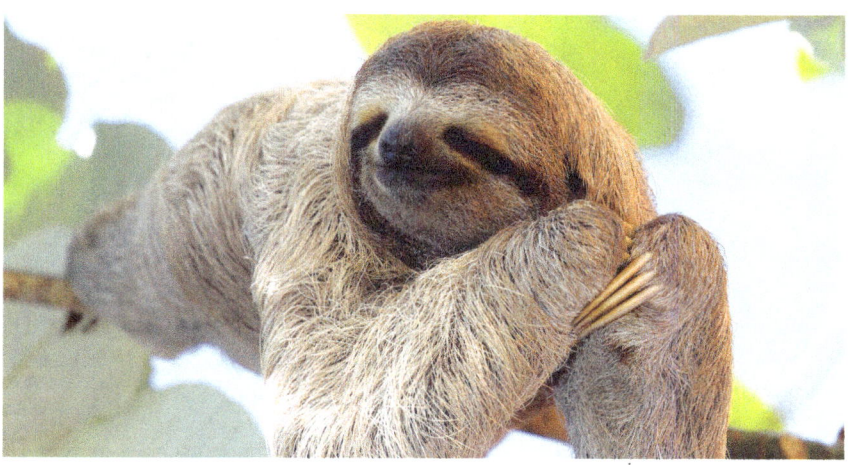

But don't sloths get a head rush from all that upside-down time? Have you ever hung upside down and felt like you might pass out? That is because when humans hang upside down, the blood rushes to our heads, and we feel faint. But sloths have developed a way to keep that from happening. Sloths have a built-in valve that doesn't allow all their blood to go to their heads when they hang upside down. So, when a sloth hangs upside down, it doesn't get dizzy and pass out. Pretty cool, right?!

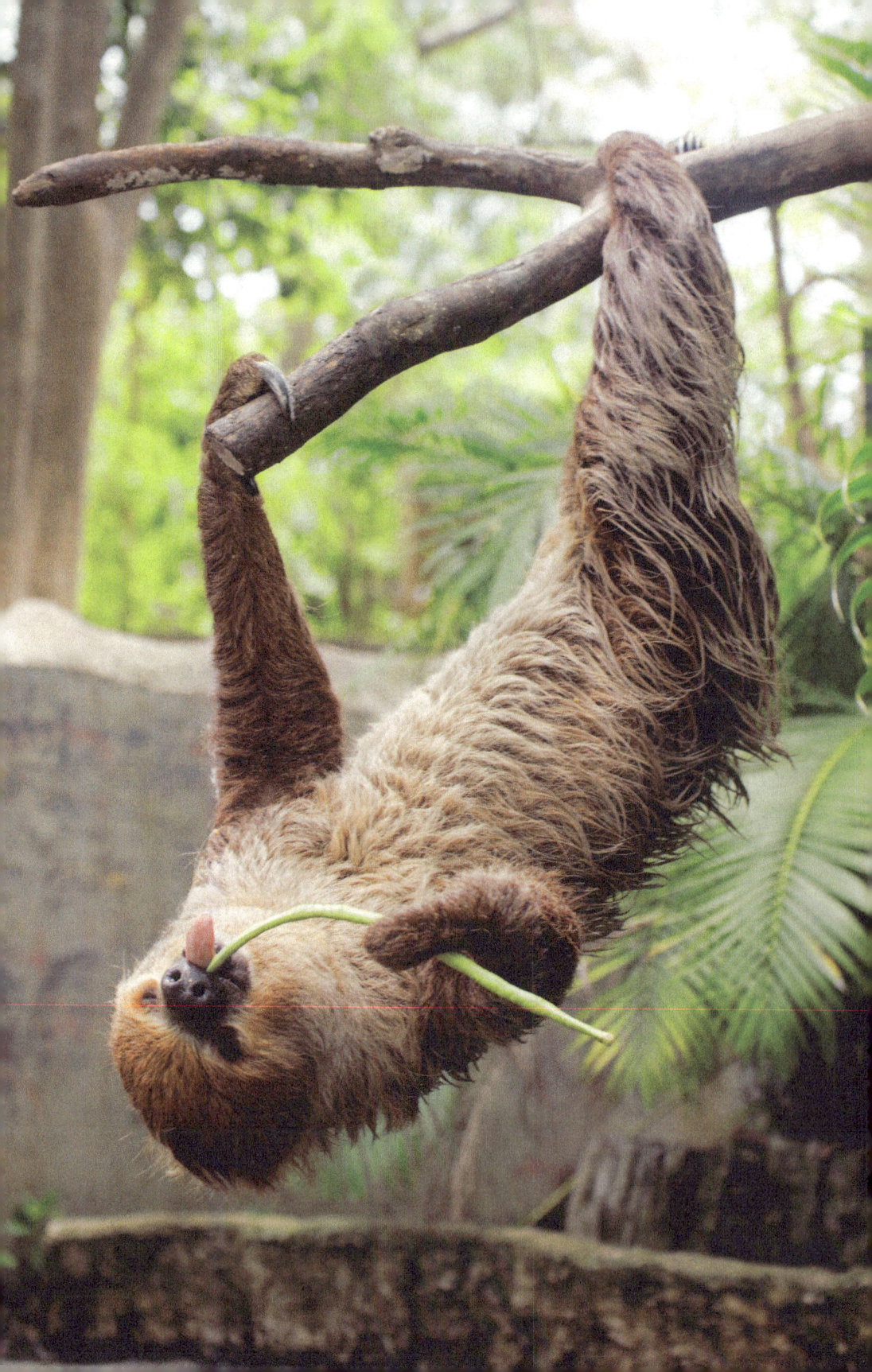

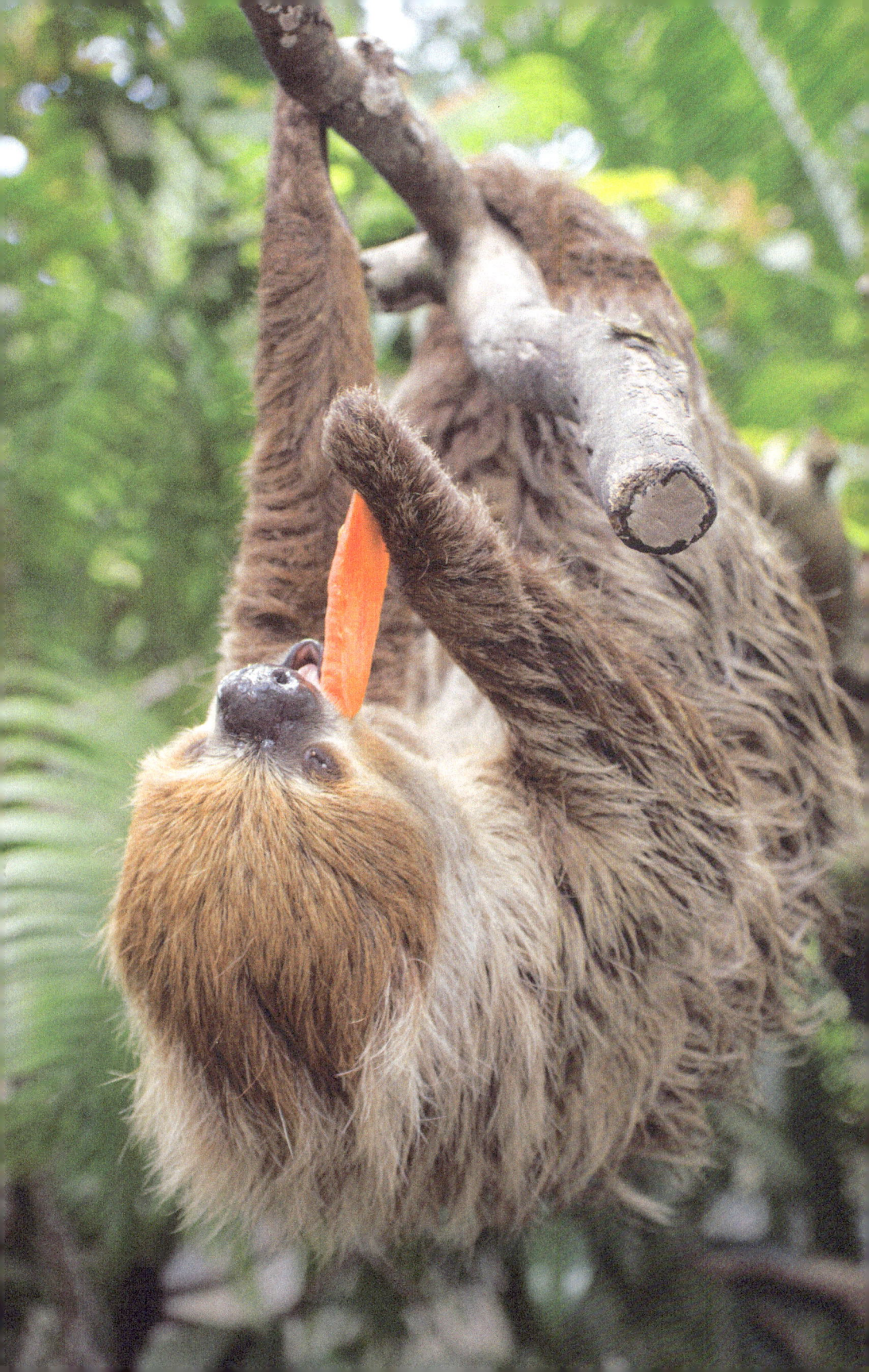

YOU'RE JUST

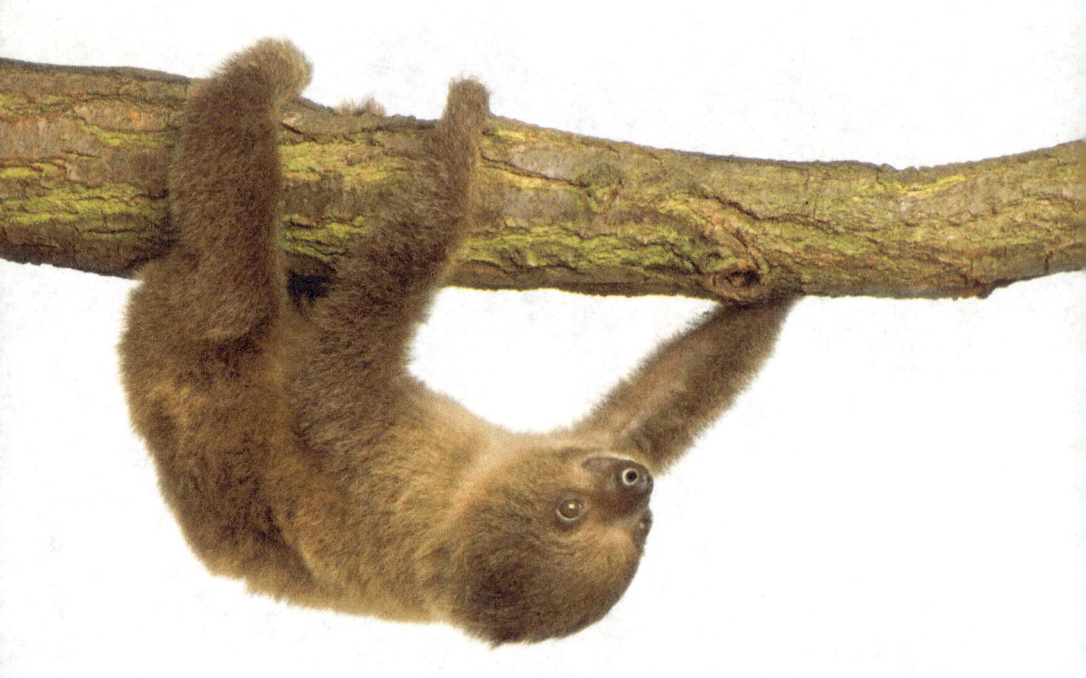

SLOTHSOME!

LIFE CYCLE

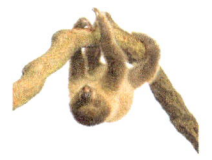

MATING

Like all mammals, the cycle of life begins for sloths when a male and female mate. Sloths can mate when they are between one and four years old, depending on the species. When they are ready to mate, female sloths let the males know through different cues.

Two-fingered sloth females send a message they are looking for a mate by rubbing their glands, found near their backside, onto the tree they live in. This way, males will smell these "*messages*" and find the female.

Three-fingered sloth females do things a little differently. Instead of leaving scented messages, these females make special sounds that are very high-pitched. Males who hear this call will come to look for the female who is in heat, which is another way of saying the female who is ready to mate.

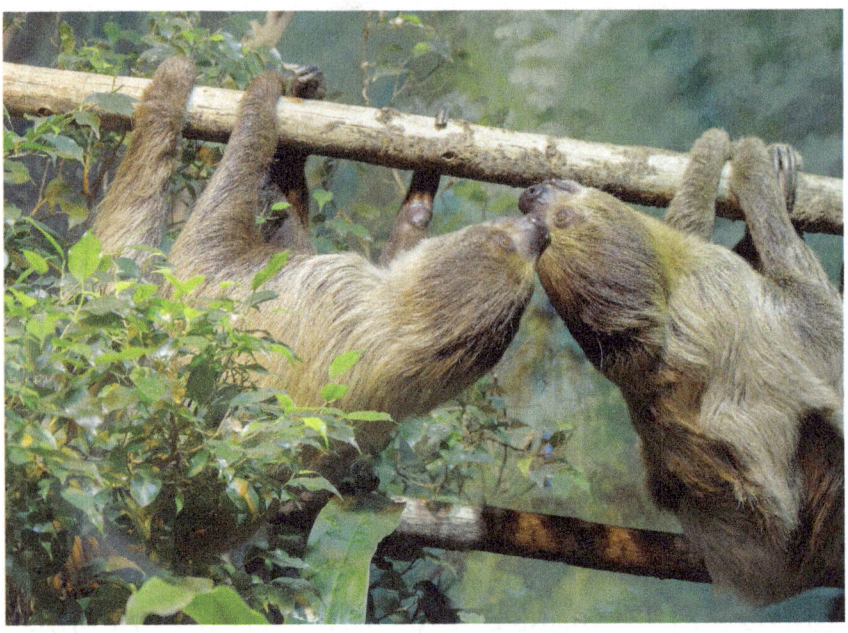

There can be trouble when more than one male sloth looks for a female. Male sloths will fight each other over the right to mate with a female. Females are not picky and will mate with as many males as they can throughout their fertile time. Sloths will fight by hanging on to each other, biting, or whacking each other with their long claws. The ultimate goal of a sloth fight is to knock the other male out of the tree. Whoever wins the sloth knock-down brawl wins the right to mate with the female. The winning male will stay with the female for several days and will also fight any other males who show up to challenge him.

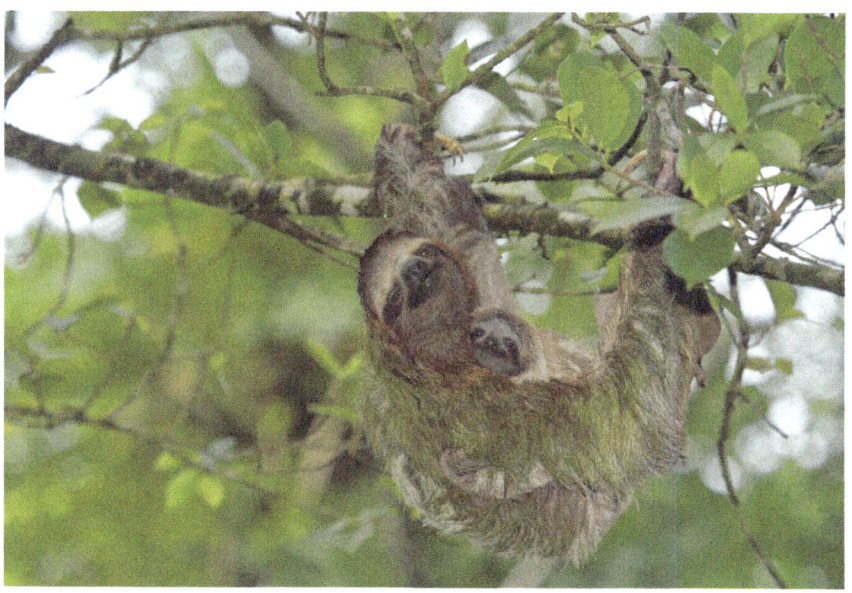

BABY SLOTHS

When a mating has been successful, a baby sloth comes onto the scene. For two-fingered sloths, females are pregnant for 11.5 months. Scientists still aren't sure how long three-fingered sloths are pregnant for, but they think it is around 6 months. Sloths give birth to a single baby at a time. While twins are possible, they are rare. As sloths only have room on their chests for one baby, they aren't able to care for both babies when twins are born. Therefore, sadly, the weaker twin will usually be abandoned.

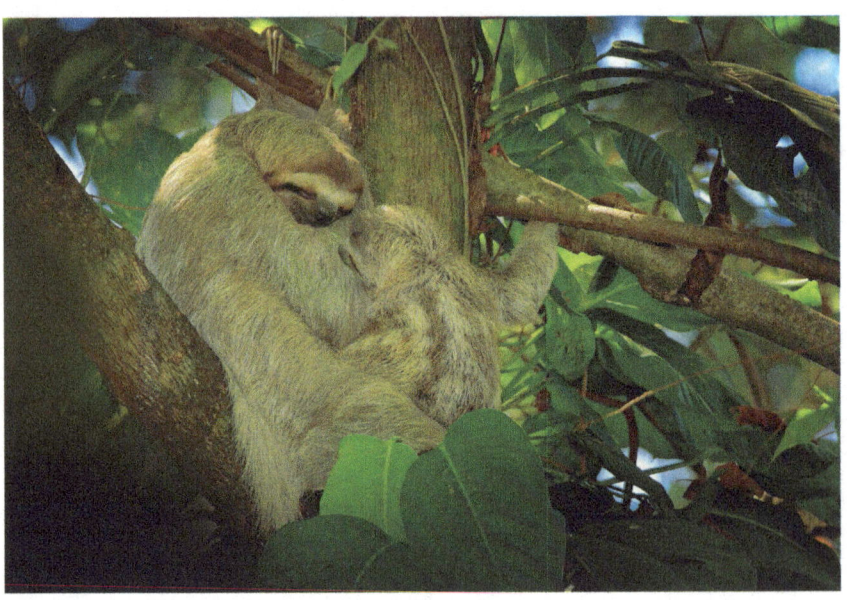

Sloths typically care for their young for 6 to 12 months, depending on the species. Just like most things sloths do, sloths give birth to their young while hanging upside down. When a female is ready to give birth, she will climb down from the higher branches to a lower spot on the tree to have her baby. This way, if the baby accidentally falls to the ground, it won't get hurt.

When a baby sloth is born, it climbs its way to its mother's chest, where it hangs on. There, it nurses from its mother for at least the next 6 months and clings to her. But as young as one week old, babies will start to taste bits of leaves from around their mother's mouth. This helps to teach them what foods and leaves are good to eat.

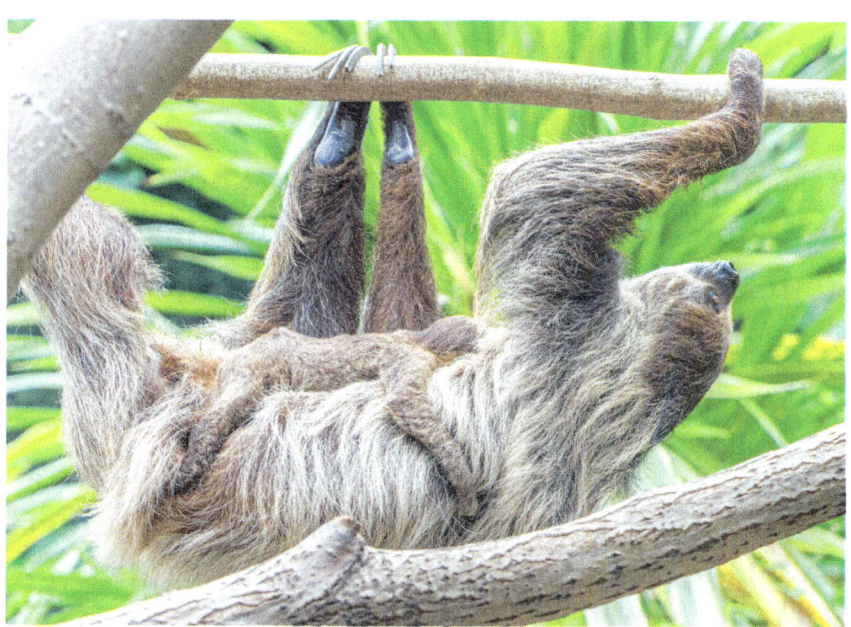

When a sloth is old enough, it will go out on its own. Sloths live alone and spend most of their lives alone, apart from the mating season.

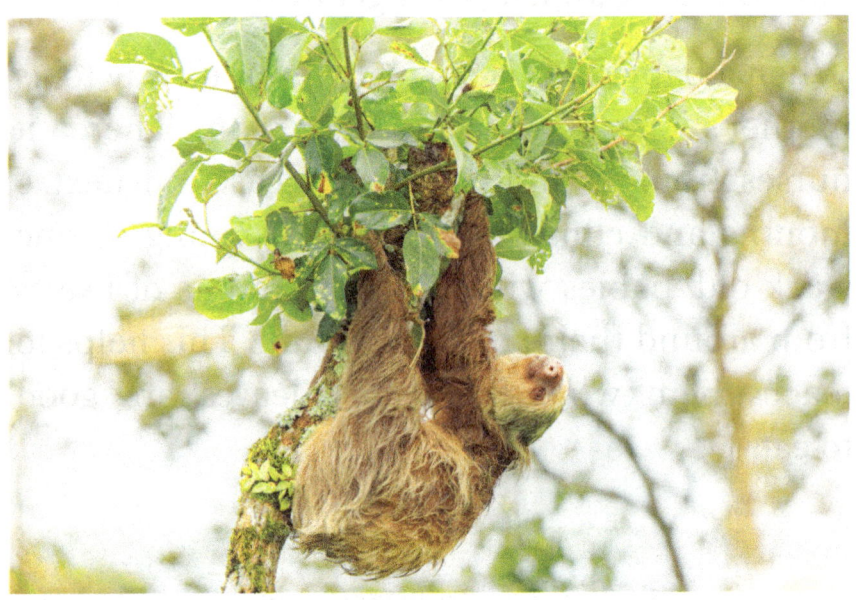

Amazingly, scientists still don't know exactly how long sloths can live. In captivity, the oldest a sloth has ever lived was 50 years. But many point out that life in captivity is very different from life in the wild.

Sloths who live in captivity seem to not move as much as sloths in the wild. The biggest difference between wild sloths and their captive versions is probably their diet. Since zoos can't replicate the tropical leaf diet of sloths, they must rely on feeding them fruits and vegetables, which the sloths cannot digest nearly as well. No one really knows what the life expectancy of a sloth might be in its natural habitat.

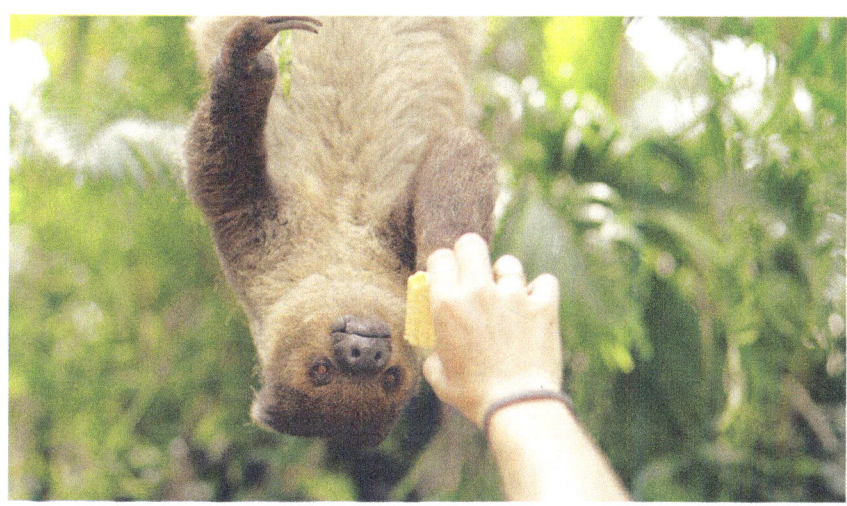

There is much room for learning more about sloths in the wild. They have proven hard to study and research in their natural environment, and many things about sloths and their behavior are still a mystery to this day. This is mainly because sloths live high up in the trees of tropical rainforests.

Who knows! Maybe one day you can study sloths and help the world learn more about these amazing creatures.

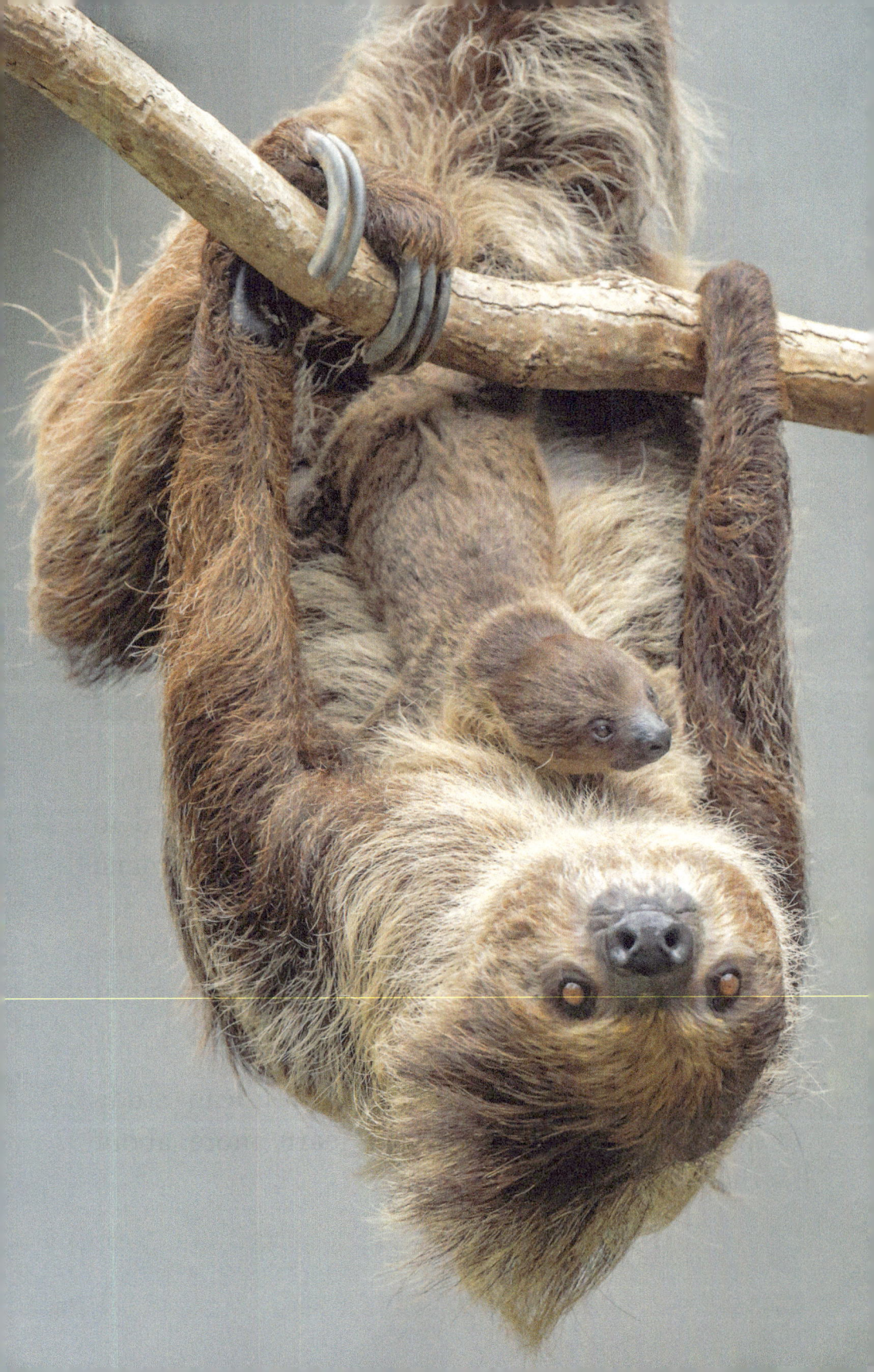

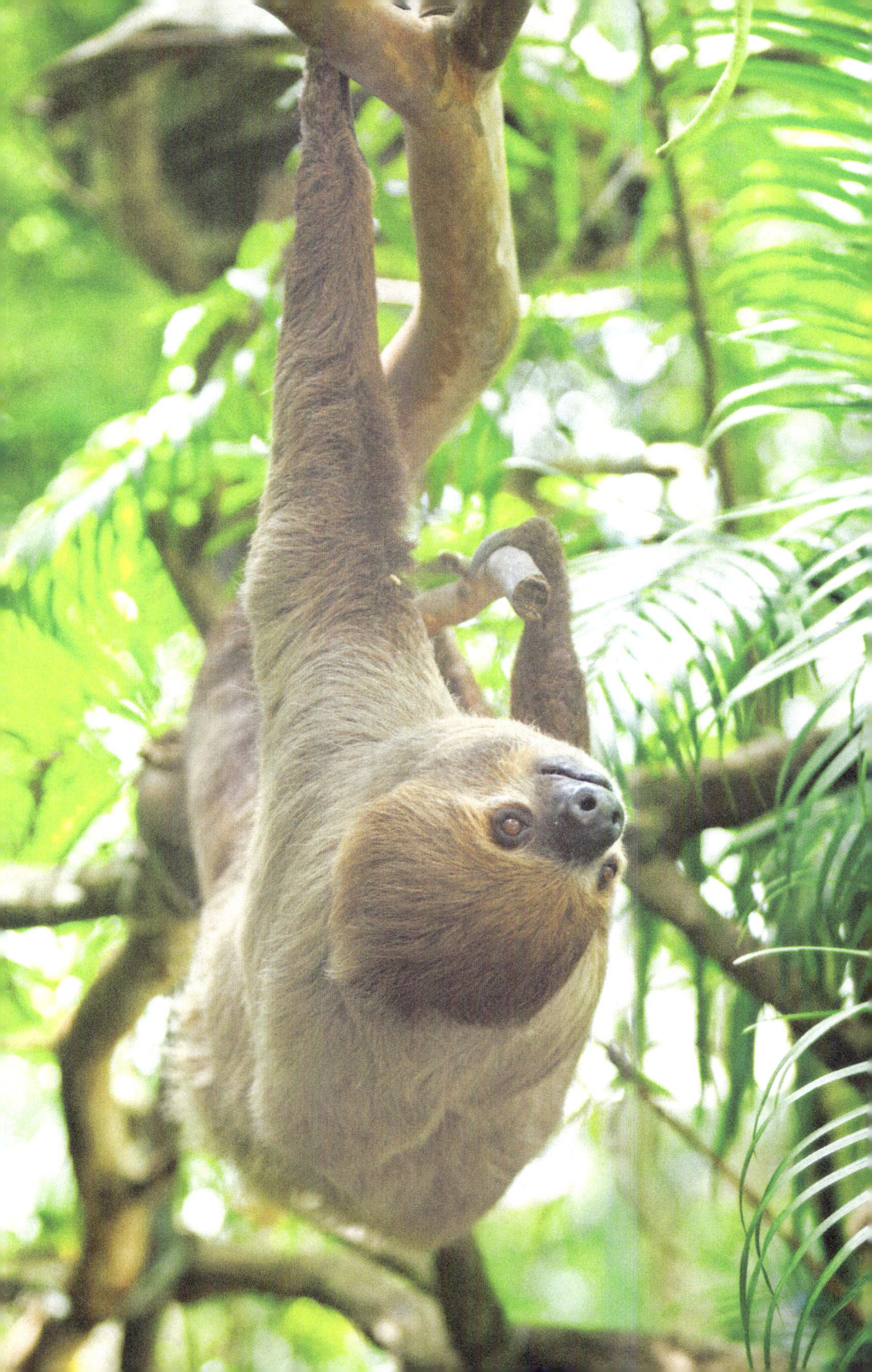

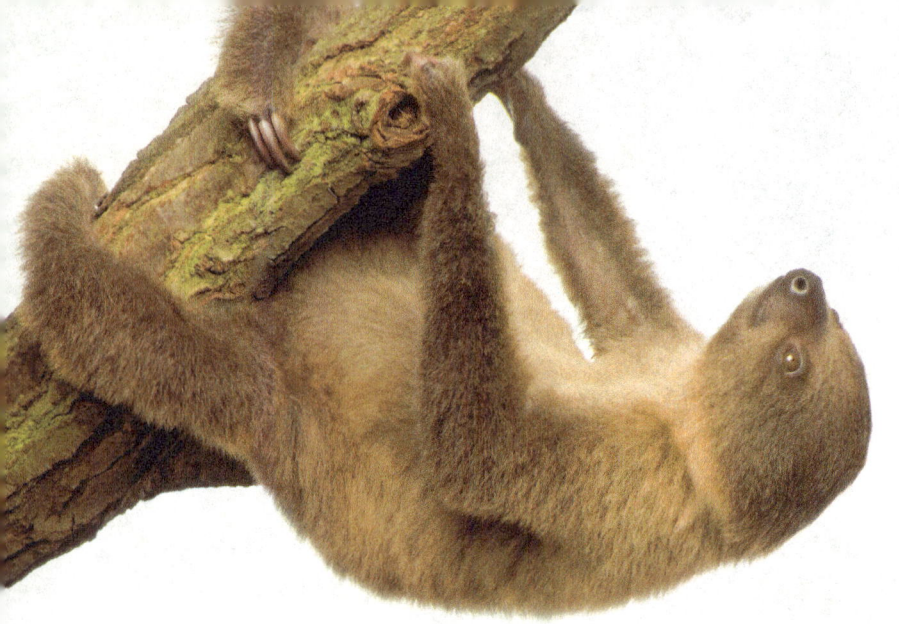

WHY ARE SLOTHS THE MOST SOCIAL ANIMALS?

Because they always wanna hang out!

MORE AWESOME FACTS

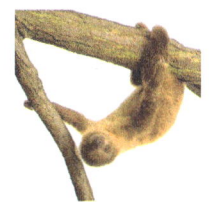

DID YOU KNOW?

- Have you ever risked your life to go to the bathroom? Sloths do this all the time! Whenever they need to poop, usually just once a week, a sloth will climb down from its tree to the forest floor. This is a dangerous place to be if you're a sloth! They may not go often, but when they do poop, they poop a lot! They can lose about 30% of their whole weight after one poop.

- Sloths have teeth and nails that grow their entire lifetime. Therefore, they can never be worn down.

- Sloths spend 90% of their time not moving at all. That means, if you had a sloth over for a sleepover and the two of you hung out for 10 hours, the sloth would move a total time of 1 hour, but for the other 9 hours, it wouldn't move at all.

- Did you know sloths are super divers? Because they can slow their heart rate down to just a third of its already slow rate, sloths can hold their breath underwater for an impressive 40 minutes! Imagine all you could see and do underwater if you could hold your breath for that long.

- Sloths don't just grow algae in their fur. Their fur can also hold beetles and other bugs. In fact, there is an entire species of moth that only lives on sloths. Scientists have found that sloth fur also holds a special kind of fungi that may be able to fight breast cancer cells!

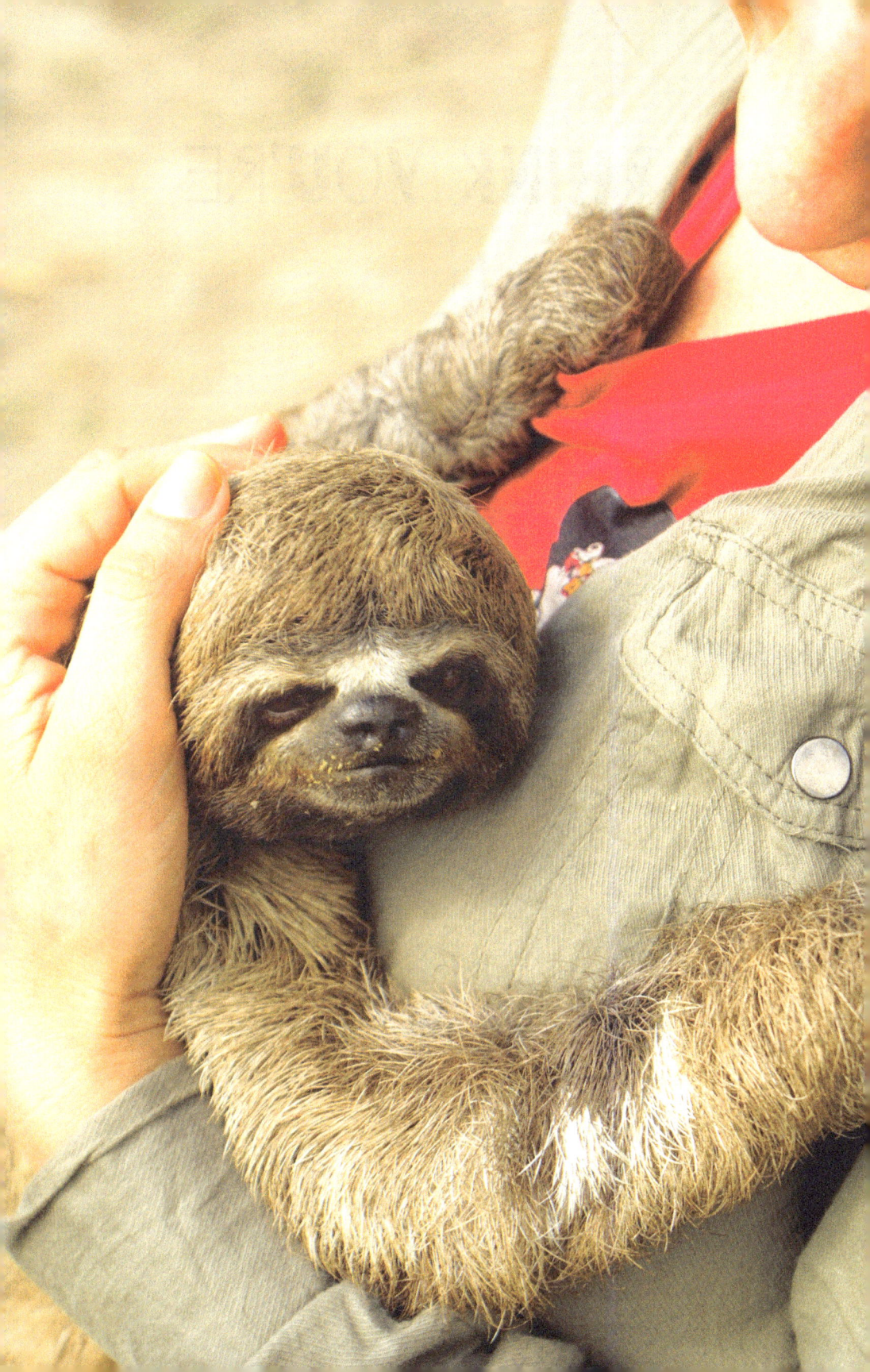

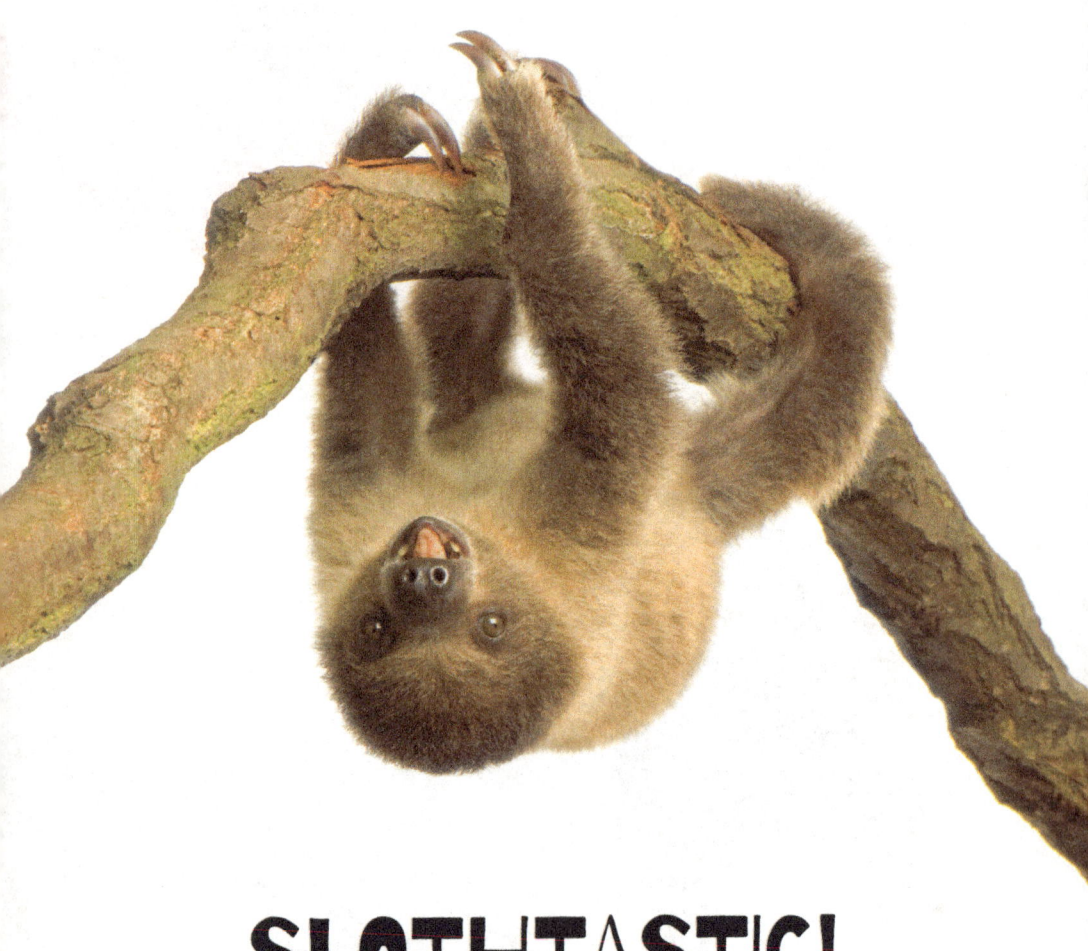

HELPING SLOTHS
THANK YOU FOR READING AND LEARNING ABOUT SLOTHS

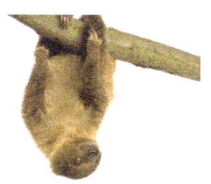

We hope you enjoyed reading about sloths and learning more about these slow-paced furry friends. Today, sloths are in danger as tropical rainforests get cut down. Thankfully, most species of sloths are quite abundant and are not endangered, but they still need people to watch out for them in this fast-paced world.

The exception is the pygmy sloth. Sadly, the pygmy sloth is currently considered to be critically endangered. Pygmy sloths only live on one small island in Panama and nowhere else in the world.

All sloths can be harmed as human activity and development gets closer and closer to their natural habitats. Something as simple as electrical wires has proven to be deadly to sloths. Natural climbers, many sloths have been hurt or killed by hanging on electrical lines and accidentally getting shocked.

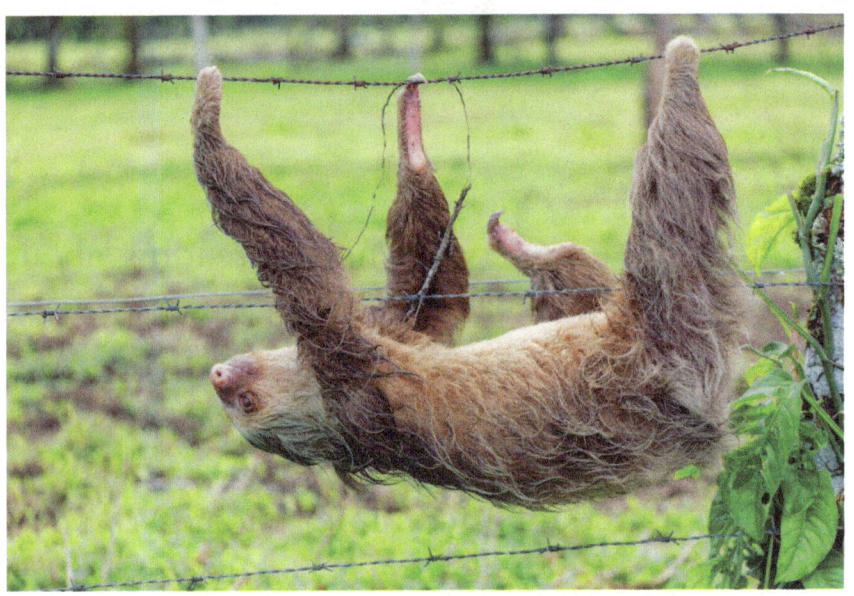

Another way sloths are harmed by humans is through poaching. Poaching is the illegal hunting of wild animals. However, thankfully hunting sloths is not very popular these days.

Humans also hurt sloths when the rainforests that the sloths live in are cut down or dwindled away. Because sloths have such specialized needs for food and shelter, they are not able to move to new areas or quickly adapt as well as some other animal species have done. We must all commit to preserving the rainforests of Central and South America. *If the rainforests are depleted, where will sloths go?*

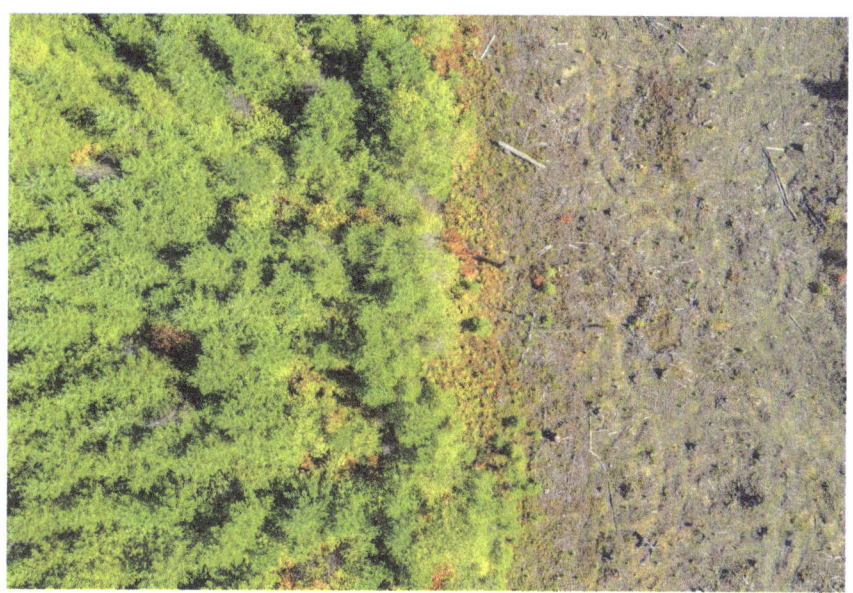

Lastly, another danger to sloths has to do with their lovable, cute looks. Sometimes, sloths are stolen from the wild and sold as pets. This is called animal trafficking. While it may seem like fun to have a sloth for a pet, sloths are wild animals that don't do well in captivity. Never buy a sloth for a pet or any wild animal. Half of the animals taken into rescue shelters in Costa Rica are sloths. Thankfully, there are organizations that work to introduce captive or kidnapped sloths back into the wild.

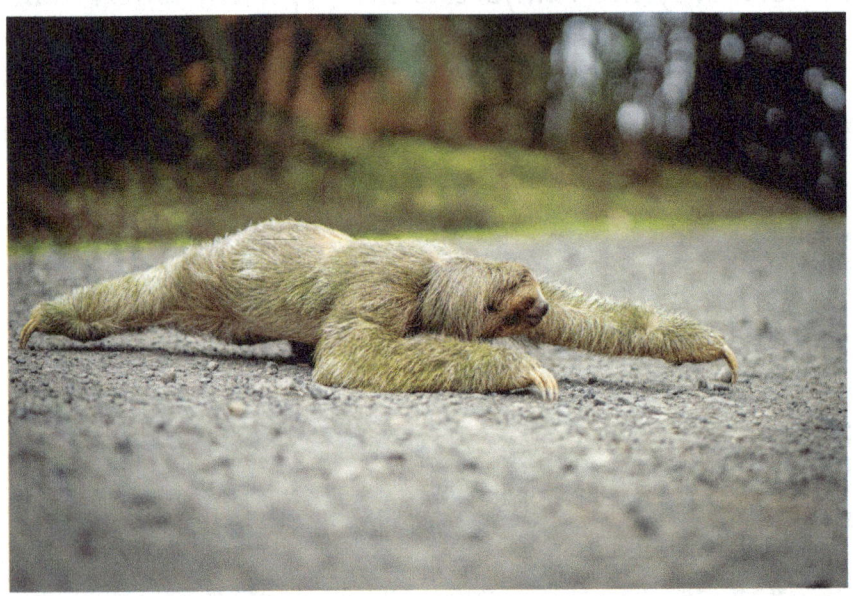

If you would like to learn more about sloths and how you can help them, check out The Sloth Conservation Foundation, which can be found at www.slothconservation.org

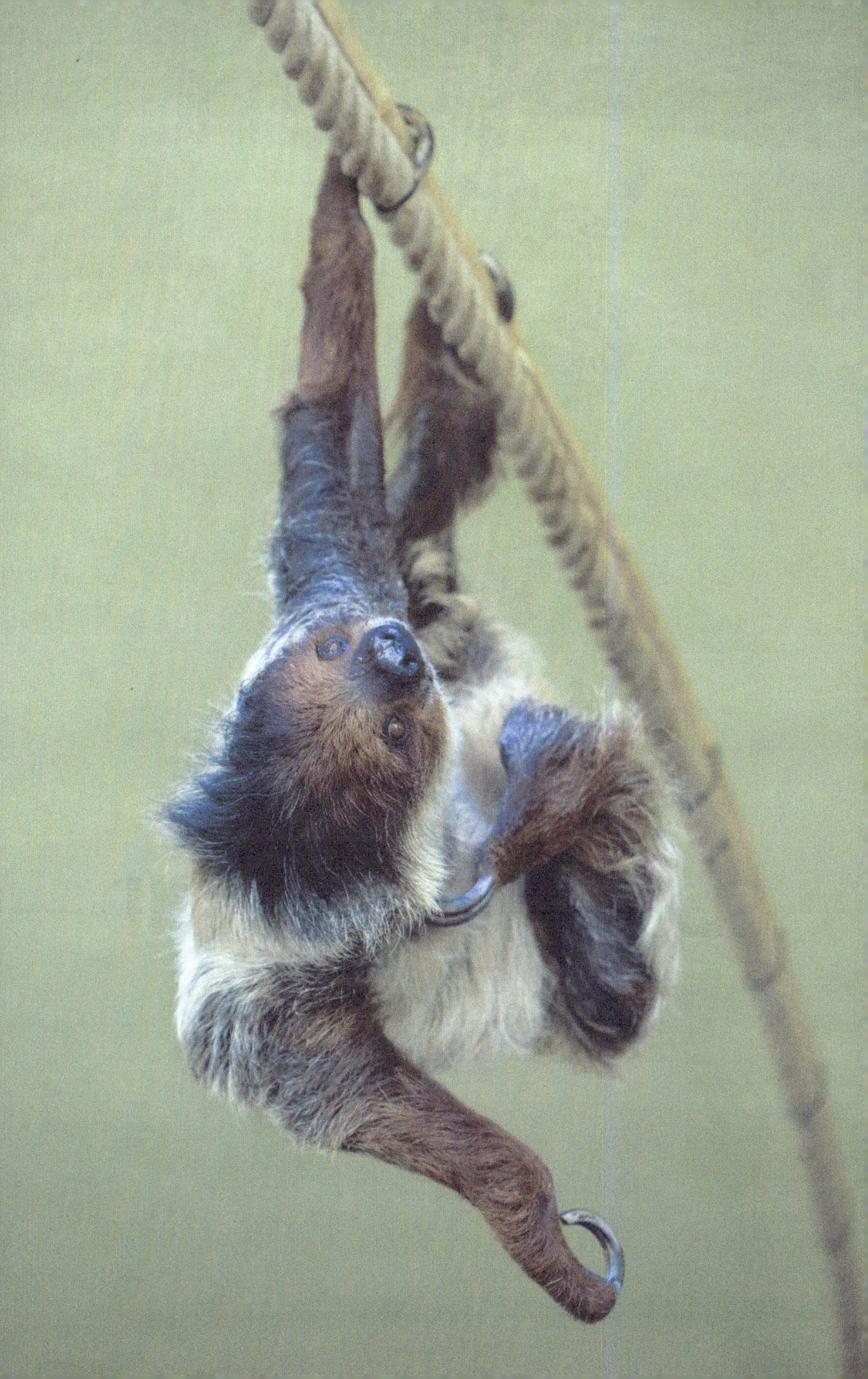

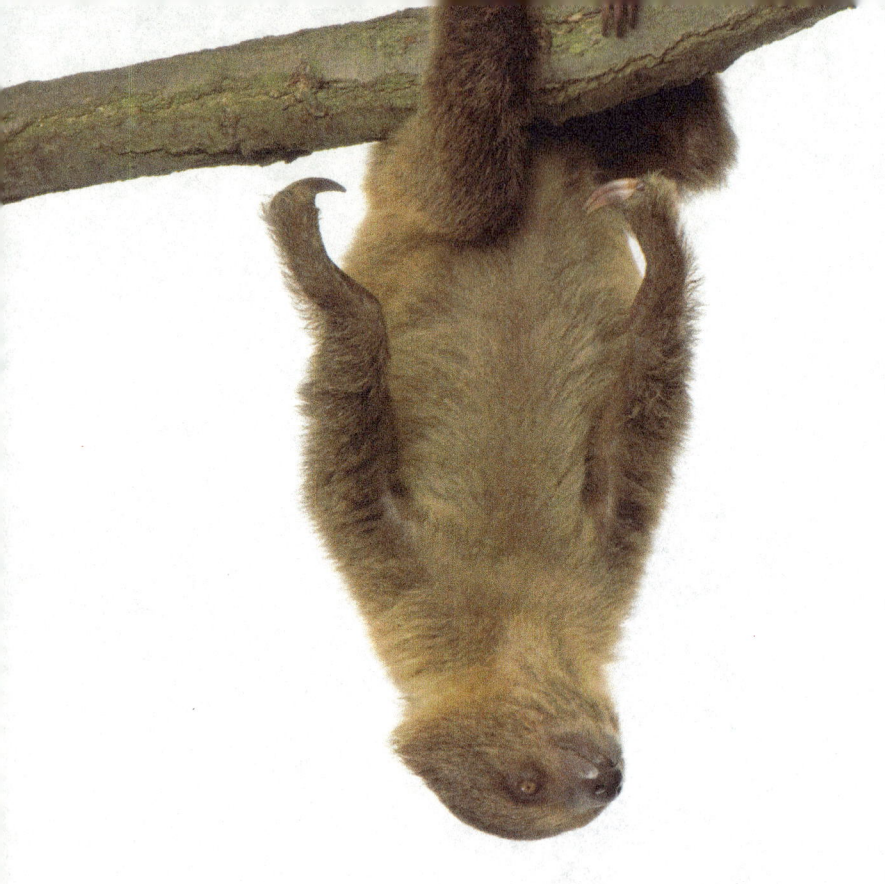

THANK YOU!

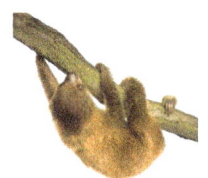

Thank you for reading this book and for allowing us to share our love for sloths with you!

If you've enjoyed this book, please let us know by leaving a rating and a brief review wherever you made your purchase! This helps us spread the word to other readers!

Thank you for your time, and have an awesome day!

For more information, please visit:

www.animalreads.com

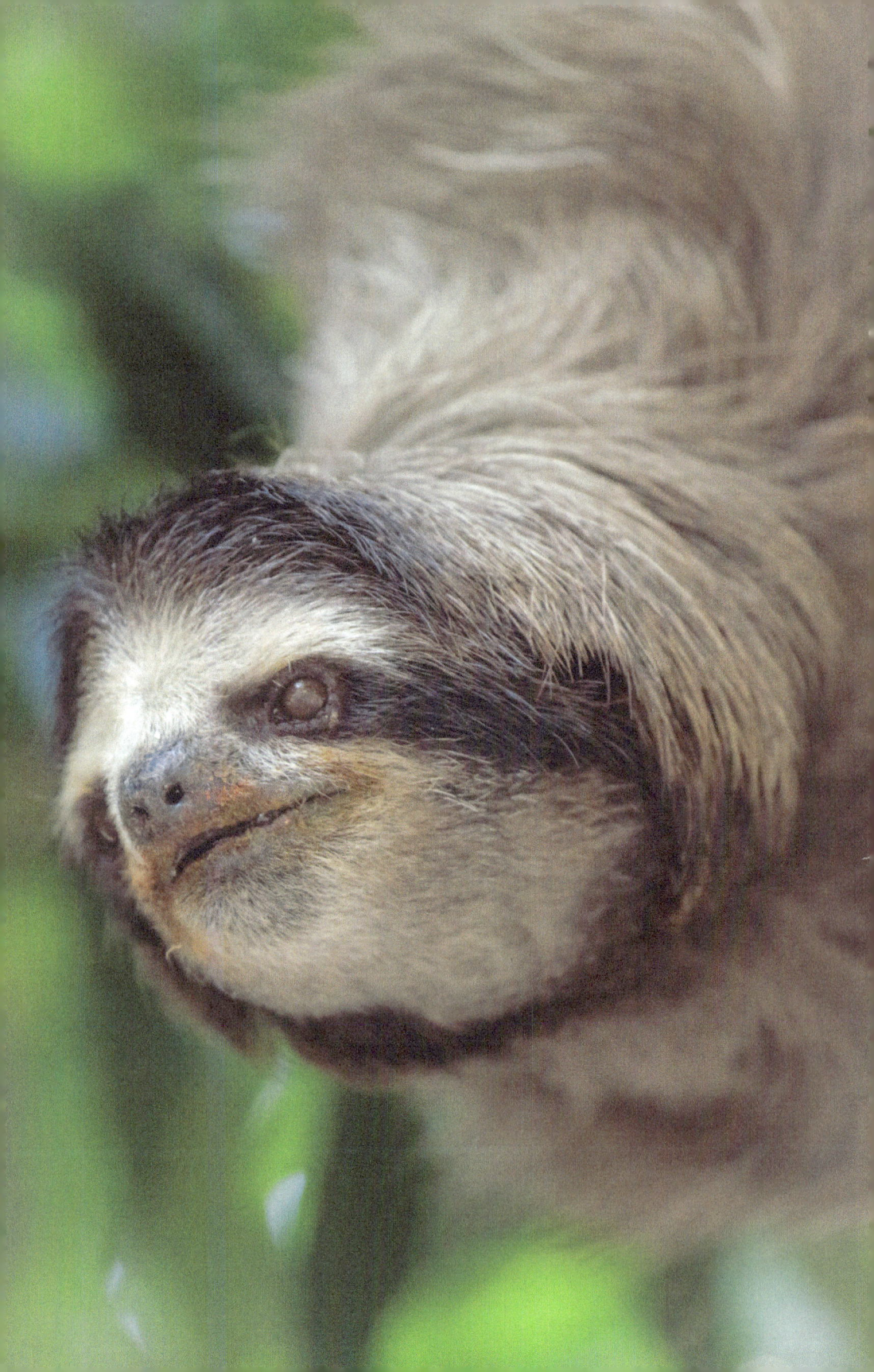

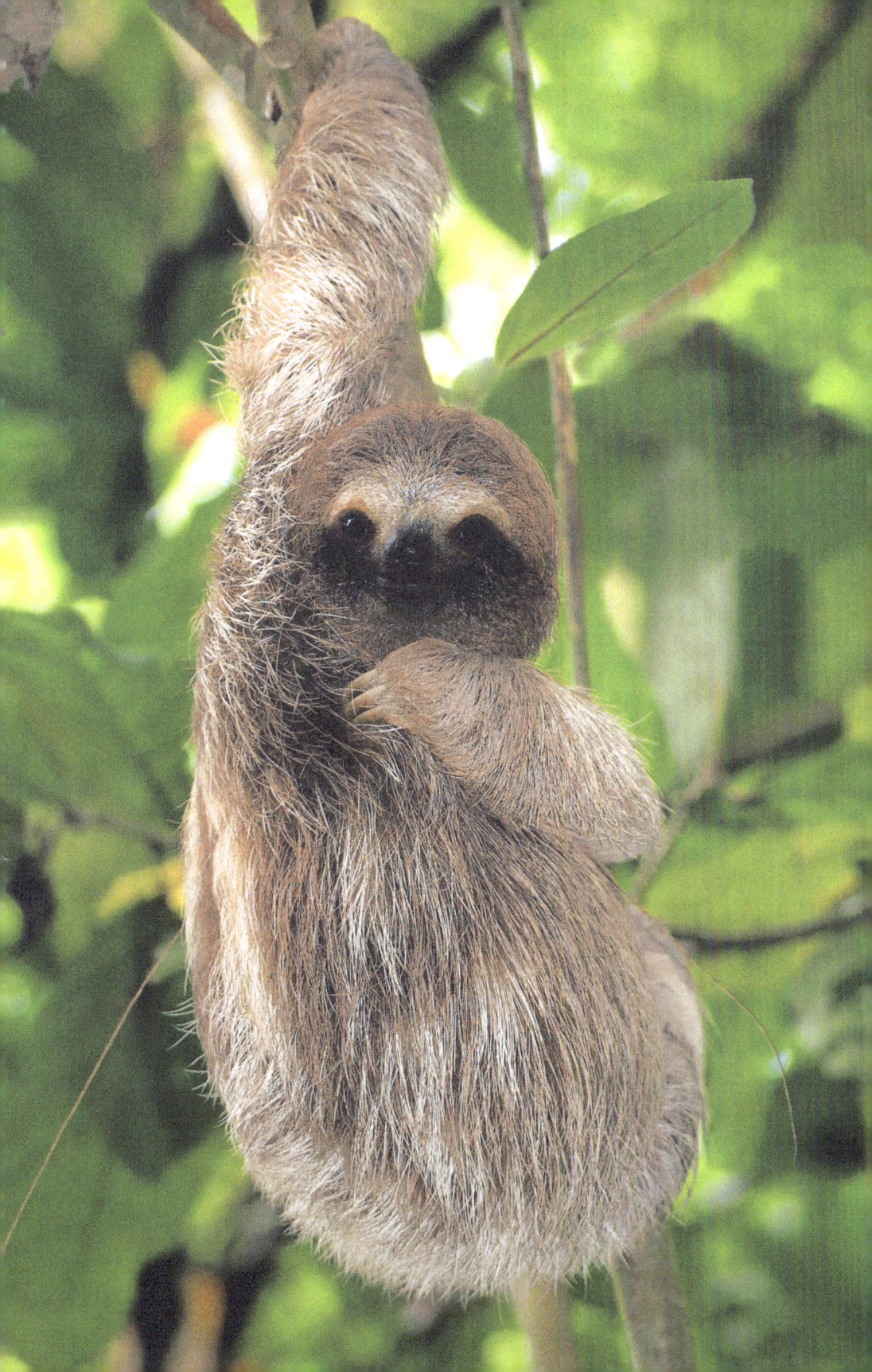

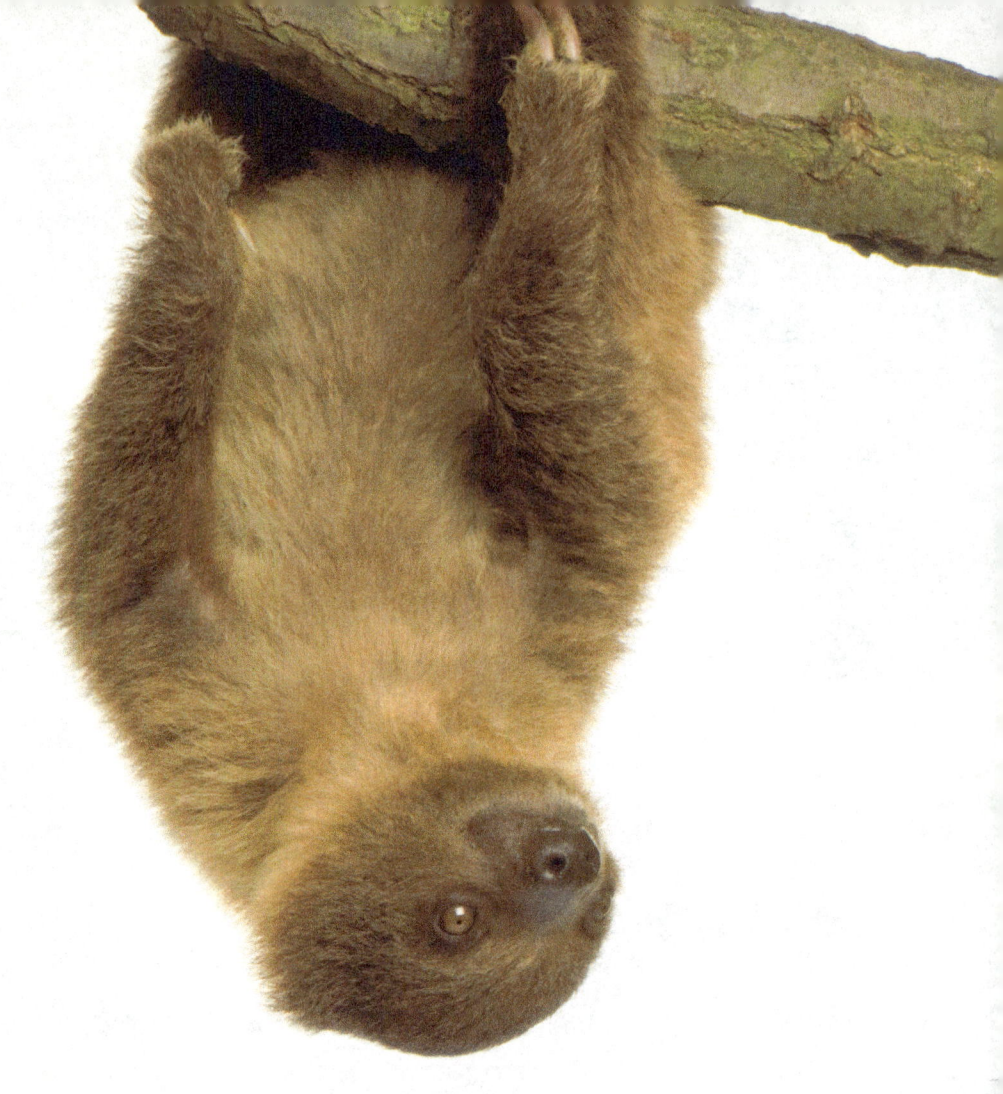

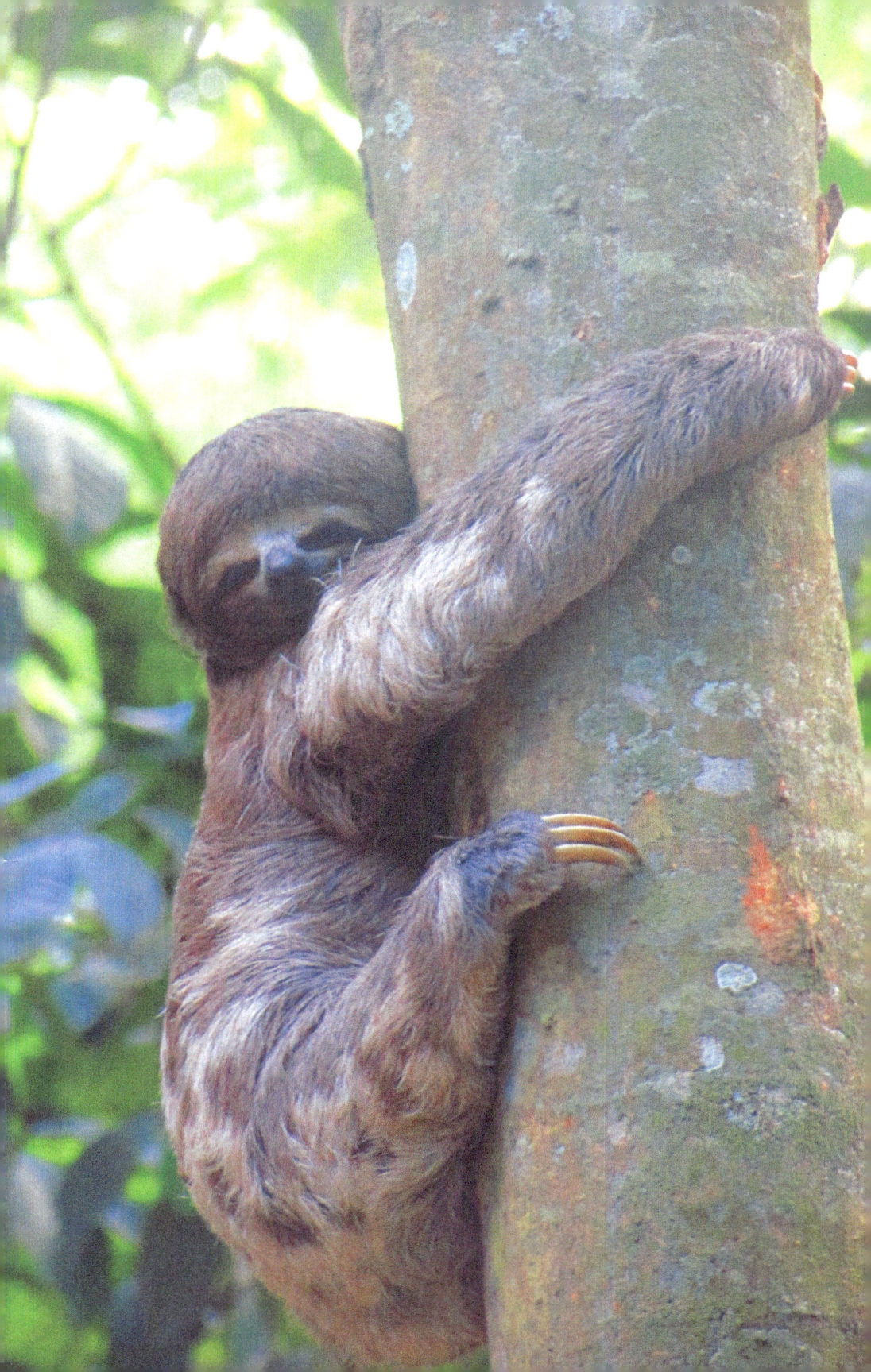

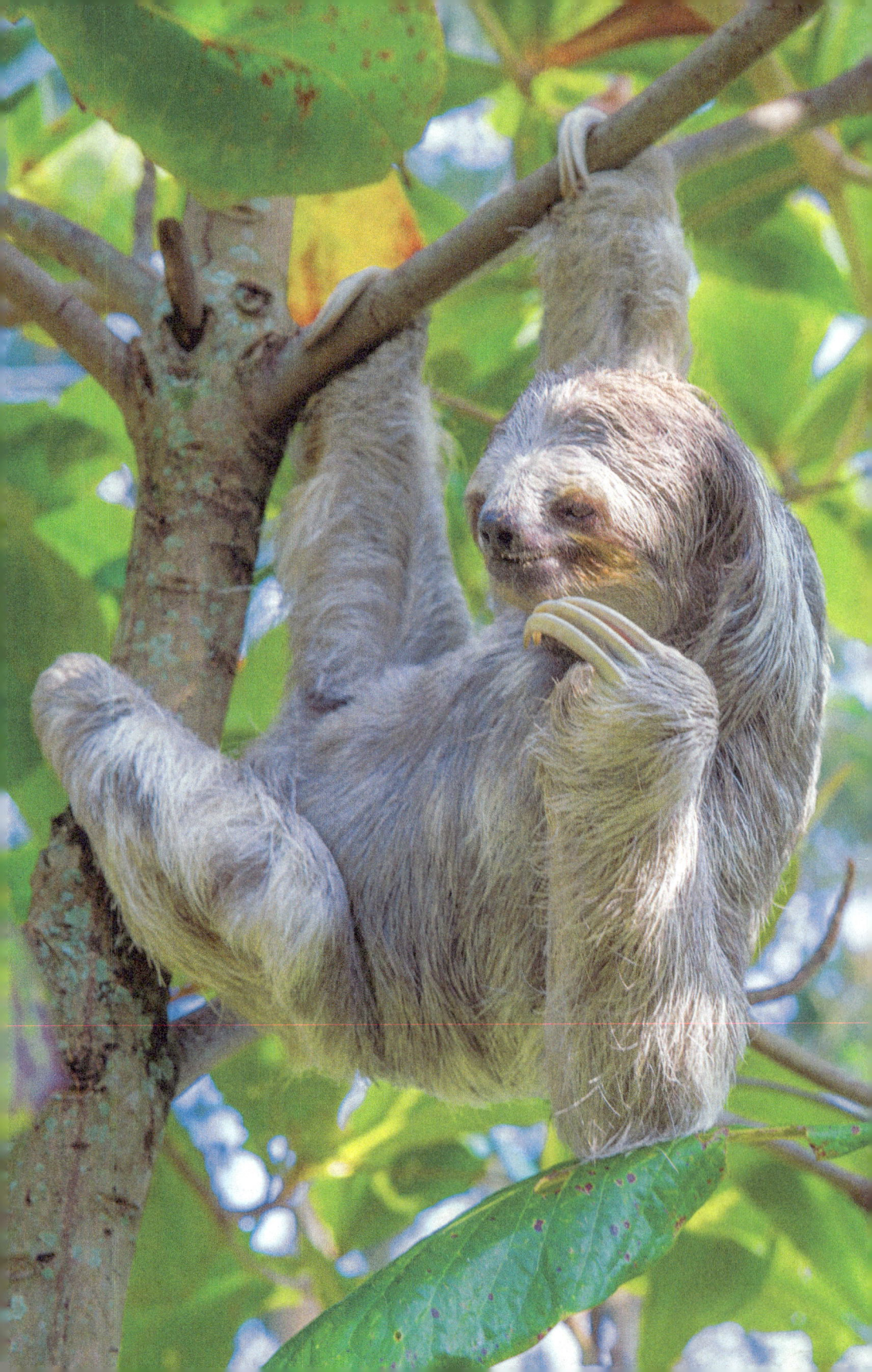

© Copyright 2022 - All rights reserved Admore Publishing

ISBN: 978-3-96772-135-5

ISBN: 978-3-96772-136-2

Animal Reads at www.animalreads.com

The content contained within this book may not be reproduced, duplicated or transmitted without direct written permission from the author or the publisher.

Under no circumstances will any blame or legal responsibility be held against the publisher, or author, for any damages, reparation, or monetary loss due to the information contained within this book. Either directly or indirectly.

Published by Admore Publishing: Gotenstraße, Berlin, Germany

www.admorepublishing.com

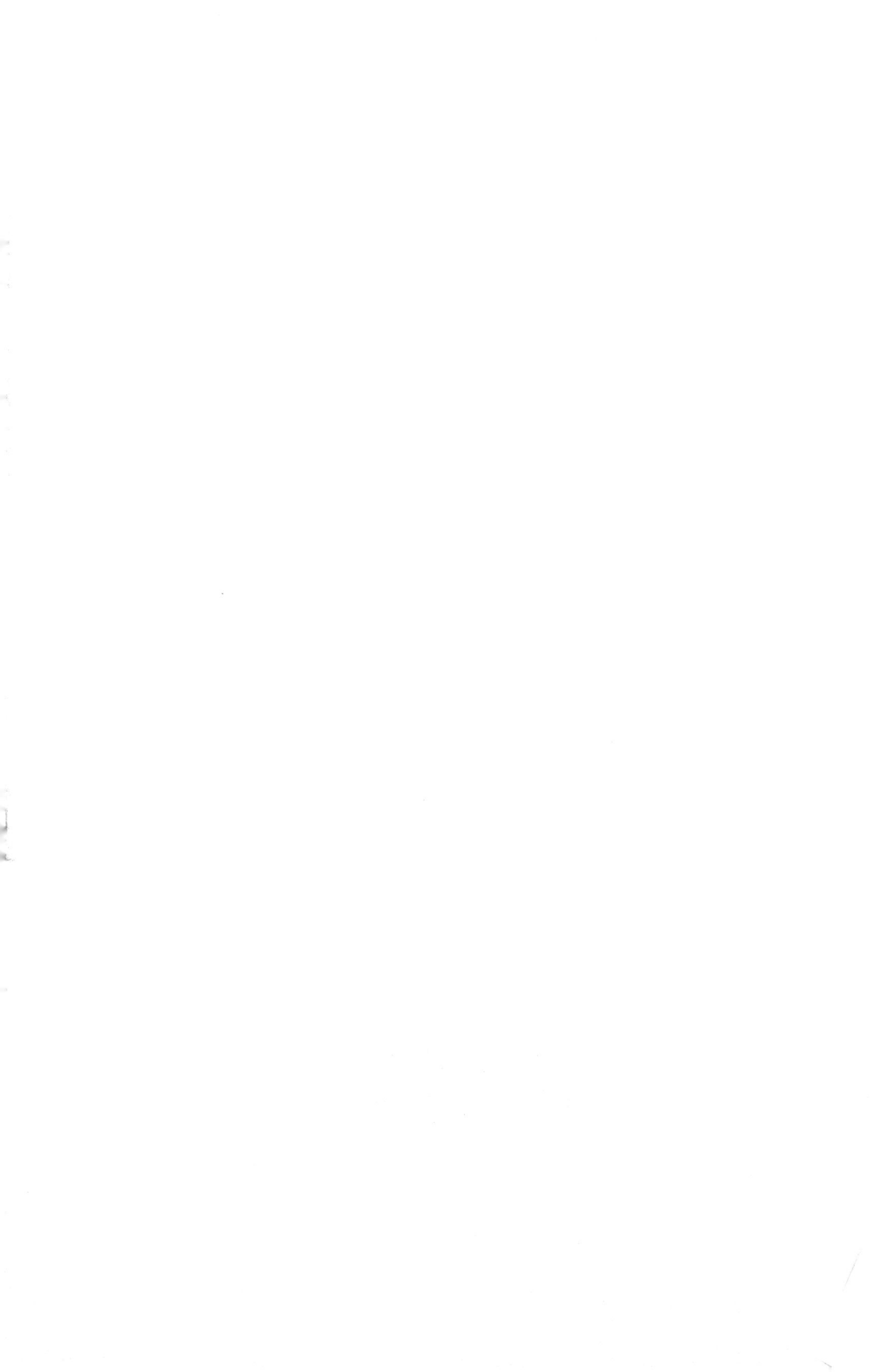

Made in the USA
Monee, IL
14 November 2024

PICTURE CREDITS

Cover: Benjavisa Ruangvaree Art/Shutterstock.com

6: Motortion Films/Shutterstock.com
10: Danita Delimont/Alamy Stock Photo
14: Sabphoto/Shutterstock.com
19: threerocksimages/Shutterstock.com
23: fizkes/Shutterstock.com
24: Faiz Zaki/Shutterstock.com
28: Ben Houdijk/Shutterstock.com
35: Just Life/Shutterstock.com
36: SDI Productions/iStock
41: Daisy Daisy/Shutterstock.com
46: Portrait Image Asia/Shutterstock.com
50: Dragon Images/Shutterstock.com
52: Pixel-Shot/Shutterstock.com

ABOUT THE AUTHOR

Carla Mooney is the author of many books for young adults and children. She lives in Pittsburgh, Pennsylvania, with her husband and three children.

as crucial to recovery, 54
  forms of, 45
  in patient-therapist relationship, 43
  peer groups, 46–47
surveys
  on mental health and COVID-19 pandemic, 7
  on stigma of mental illness in workplace, 27
  on use of online resources on mental illness, 26

This Is My Brave, 31
Tracy, Natasha, 31
treatment(s)
  animal therapy, 51–54
  art therapy, 49–50
  cognitive behavioral therapy, 5, 35–37
  cost as barrier to, 42
  dialectical behavioral therapy, 37–38
  electroconvulsive therapy, 13
  medication, 34, 40–41
  percentage of youth with depression not receiving, 33
  psychotherapy, 34–35
  stigma as barrier to seeking, 22–23, 28, 30–31
trichotillomania, 36–37

Wick, Claire, 53
Wright, Kayla, 37–38

yoga, 47–48

Kaiser Family Foundation, 6
Keenmon, Corinna, 48
Kraus, Jen, 51–52

Lady Gaga, 27
Lovato, Demi, 27–28, **28**

Malkin, Vicky, 42–43
Martino, Angela, 51–52
McIntyre, Phil, 28
medications, psychiatric, 34, 40–41
meditation, 48
Mental Health America, 6, 33, 58
mental health disorders
   associated with substance abuse, 12
   impacts on career/finances, 12–15
   physical effects of, 12
   prevalence of, 6, 11
   relationships strained by, 16–18, **19**
   risky behaviors and, 18–20
   school difficulties and, 15–16
   suicide associated with, 34
   types of, 6
   warning signs of, 17
   See also treatment(s)
Murthy, Vivek, 7

National Alliance on Mental Illness (NAMI), 11, 12, 34, 58
National Council for Mental Wellbeing, 42
National Institute of Mental Health (NIMH), 59
National Suicide Prevention Lifeline, 59
NITEO program (Boston University), 16
Noonan, Susan, 17–18

norepinephrine, 40

opinion polls. *See* surveys

Phelps, Michael, 27
physical ailments
   mental illness and risks for, 12
   as warning sign, 17
polls. *See* surveys
post-traumatic stress disorder (PTSD)
   prevalence of, 11
   treatment of, 38–39, 51, 53, 54
psychotherapy, 34–35

schizoaffective disorder, 48
schizophrenia, 36, 40, 48
self-care, forms of, 47–49
self-harm behaviors, 18–19
serotonin, 40
Spot to Talk clinic, 53
Srivastava, Varsha, 15–16
Stein, Joshua David, 32–33
stigma, 23
   as barrier to seeking treatment, 22–23, 28
   cultural influences on, 24–26
   media portrayal of mental illness and, 24
   in workplace, 27
Substance Abuse and Mental Health Services Administration (SAMHSA), 59
substance abuse/use, 51
   associated with mental health disorders, 12
   as attempt to self-medicate, 18
   as warning sign, 17
suicide, 17, 34, 46
Super, Nora, 9
support/support systems, 8, 29
   animal therapy and, 51–53

INDEX

Note: Boldface page numbers indicate illustrations.

American Psychiatric Association, 22–23, 27, 58
American Psychological Association, 58
animal therapy, 51–54
anxiety disorder, 44, 47
   medications for, 40
   prevalence of, 11
   therapy for, 35–36
art therapy, 49–50

Barge, David, 39
Bean, Sara, 29
bipolar disorder
   medications for, 40
   prevalence of, 11
borderline personality disorder, 33
Boston University, 16
Brandoff, Rachel, 50
Brown, Jamie, 29

Centers for Disease Control and Prevention (CDC), 58
cognitive behavioral therapy (CBT), 5, 35–37
Cohen Veterans Network, 42
COVID-19 pandemic, 7
Cruwys, Tegan, 54
cutting, 19–20

de Blasio, Bill, 6–7
depression, 4, 21–22, 26, 50
   antidepressant therapy for, 40
   hospitalization for, 45–46
   percentage of affected youth not receiving treatment, 33
   prevalence of, 11
   recurrence of, 10–11
   risky behaviors and, 18–19
dialectical behavioral therapy (DBT), 37–38
dogs, emotional support, 53–54
dopamine, 40

eating well, 48
electroconvulsive therapy (ECT), 13
endorphins, 18–19, 47
equine therapy, 51–52, **52**, 53
exercise, 47, 48–49
exposure therapy, 39–40
eye movement desensitization and reprocessing (EMDR) therapy, 38–39

Face It (support group), 46

gamma-aminobutyric acid, 48

Hall, Will, 48–49
Hark, Danielle, 50
Hertzog, Chelsea, 44, 45
Hewlett, Finlaey, 54
hospitalization, 38, 45–46

Johnson, Dwayne, 27
Joker (film), 24
Joly-Lowdermilk, Courtney, 16
Jonas, Joe, 28
Jonas, Nick, 28

FOR FURTHER RESEARCH

Books

A.W. Buckey, *Dealing with Anxiety Disorder*. San Diego, CA: ReferencePoint, 2020.

Matt Chandler, *Understanding Mental Health*. Ann Arbor, MI: Cherry Lake, 2020.

Tabatha Chansard, *Conquer Anxiety Workbook for Teens: Find Peace from Worry, Panic, Fear, and Phobias*. Emeryville, CA: Althea, 2019.

Elisabeth Herschbach, *Teens and Mental Health*. San Diego, CA: ReferencePoint, 2019.

Nadra Nittle, *America's Mental Health Crisis*. New York: Greenhaven, 2020.

Barbara Sheen, *Teen Guide to Managing Stress and Anxiety*. San Diego, CA: ReferencePoint, 2022.

Internet Sources

Dani Blum and Farah Miller, "How to Improve Your Mental Health in 2022," *New York Times*, December 30, 2021. www.nytimes.com.

Michele C. Hollow, "Fighting the Stigma of Mental Illness Through Music," *New York Times*, January 29, 2019. www.nytimes.com.

Mental Health America, "The State of Mental Health in America," 2021. https://mhanational.org.

NIH Medline Plus Magazine, "Reaching Great Heights with Anxiety and Depression," November 5, 2019. https://magazine.medlineplus.gov.

US Department of Health and Human Services, "Protecting Youth Mental Health: The U.S. Surgeon General's Advisory," 2021. www.hhs.gov.

Venus Williams, "Venus Williams: The Thing That Has Really Made Me Tough," *New York Times*, September 11, 2021. www.nytimes.com.

National Institute of Mental Health (NIMH)
www.nimh.nih.gov

The NIMH is the federal government's chief funding agency for mental health research in America. The institute's website provides a variety of information and fact sheets on mental health disorders, treatments, and the latest mental health research.

National Suicide Prevention Lifeline
https://suicidepreventionlifeline.org
1 (800) 273-8255

The National Suicide Prevention Lifeline is a national network of local crisis centers. It operates around the clock and provides free and confidential support for people experiencing a suicidal crisis or emotional distress.

Substance Abuse and Mental Health Services Administration (SAMHSA) National Helpline
www.samhsa.gov/find-help/national-helpline
1 (800) 662-4357

SAMHSA is an agency in the US Department of Health and Human Services that works to reduce the impact of substance abuse and mental illness in America. It operates an around-the-clock help line for people facing mental or substance use disorders.

GETTING HELP AND INFORMATION

American Psychiatric Association
www.psychiatry.org
The American Psychiatric Association is an organization of member physicians working together to ensure humane care and effective treatment for all persons with mental disorders. Its website includes a special section on mental health resources for families.

American Psychological Association
www.apa.org
The American Psychological Association represents American psychologists who study and treat human behavior. The association's website features information and resources for psychologists, health care workers, and the general public about various mental health topics.

Centers for Disease Control and Prevention (CDC)
www.cdc.gov
The CDC is the premier public health agency in the United States. Its website includes the latest information about mental health disorders, treatment, and research.

Mental Health America
www.mhanational.org
Mental Health America is an advocacy group for people with mental illnesses and their families. Its website features many resources, including an interactive tool to assist in finding mental health help, information on support groups, and mental health screening tools.

National Alliance on Mental Illness (NAMI)
www.nami.org
The NAMI is an advocacy group for people with mental illnesses and has local chapters across the country. Its website offers a variety of resources, including information about mental health conditions, support groups, help lines, and more.

41. David Barge, "EMDR Therapy Transformed My Life," Welldoing.org, September 5, 2019. https://welldoing.org.
42. Barge, "EMDR Therapy Transformed My Life."
43. Lily Burana, "My Mental Health Issues Have a Name: Bruce," *New York Times*, October 14, 2021. www.nytimes.com.
44. Vicky Malkin, "My Journey with Therapy and Chronic Depression," Welldoing.org, July 12, 2018. https://welldoing.org.
45. Malkin, "My Journey with Therapy and Chronic Depression."
46. Malkin, "My Journey with Therapy and Chronic Depression."

Chapter Four: Lifelong Strategies

47. Chelsea Hertzog, "How Music Gives Me Hope in My Mental Illness Recovery," The Mighty, May 2, 2017. https://themighty.com.
48. Hertzog, "How Music Gives Me Hope in My Mental Illness Recovery."
49. Hertzog, "How Music Gives Me Hope in My Mental Illness Recovery."
50. Al, "Success Story: Al," Face It Foundation, 2022. www.faceitfoundation.org.
51. Al, "Success Story."
52. Quoted in Theresa Tamkins, "19 Moving Stories from People Who Used Exercise to Change Their Life," BuzzFeed News, January 16, 2019. www.buzzfeednews.com.
53. Quoted in Patti Muck, "The Benefits of Yoga: How It Boosts Your Mental Health," *Tips to Live By* (blog), Houston Methodist, September 14, 2021. www.houstonmethodist.org.
54. Will Hall, "Will Hall's Recovery Story," National Empowerment Center, 2022. https://power2u.org.
55. Quoted in Aneri Pattani, "How Creative Arts Can Change the Way People Deal with Mental Illness," *Philadelphia (PA) Inquirer*, November 5, 2018. www.inquirer.com.
56. Quoted in Pattani, "How Creative Arts Can Change the Way People Deal with Mental Illness."
57. Quoted in Pattani, "How Creative Arts Can Change the Way People Deal with Mental Illness."
58. Quoted in Mary Carole McCauley, "Equine-Assisted Therapy in Harford Helps Improve Mental Health Through Interaction and Activity," *Baltimore (MD) Sun*, February 25, 2021. www.baltimoresun.com.
59. Quoted in McCauley, "Equine-Assisted Therapy in Harford Helps Improve Mental Health Through Interaction and Activity."
60. Quoted in Touchstone Mental Health, "Simone's Story," 2017. www.touchstonemh.org.
61. Quoted in Lucy Sweeney and Dariya Salmin, "Young People Are Struggling the Most with Their Mental Health. Here's What They've Learned from Asking for Help," ABC News, June 8, 2021. www.abc.net.au.
62. Quoted in Sweeney and Salmin, "Young People Are Struggling the Most with Their Mental Health."

17. Quoted in Tugend, "A Climb Out of Depression, Doubt and Academic Failure."
18. Susan Noonan, "Mental Illness Splits Families," *View the Mist* (blog), *Psychology Today*, May 18, 2017. www.psychologytoday.com.
19. Quoted in Benedict Carey, "Getting a Handle on Self-Harm," *New York Times*, November 11, 2019. www.nytimes.com.
20. Quoted in Carey, "Getting a Handle on Self-Harm."

Chapter Two: Overcoming the Stigma of Mental Illness

21. Vic, "Vic's Story," Make It OK. https://makeitok.org.
22. Vic, "Vic's Story."
23. Vic, "Vic's Story."
24. Quoted in Deconstructing Stigma, "Ramya," 2022. https://deconstructingstigma.org.
25. Quoted in Deconstructing Stigma, "Ramya."
26. Quoted in Deconstructing Stigma, "Ramya."
27. Quoted in Deconstructing Stigma, "Dominique," 2022. https://deconstructingstigma.org.
28. Quoted in Deconstructing Stigma, "Dominique."
29. Quoted in Colby Itkowitz, "Demi Lovato Lives with Bipolar Disorder. Before Every Concert, She Holds Mental-Health Workshops for Fans," *Washington Post*, July 27, 2016. www.washingtonpost.com.
30. Quoted in Luna Greenstein, "9 Ways to Fight Mental Health Stigma," National Alliance on Mental Illness, October 11, 2017. www.nami.org.
31. Quoted in Greenstein, "9 Ways to Fight Mental Health Stigma."
32. Quoted in Deconstructing Stigma, "Marilyn," 2022. https://deconstructingstigma.org.
33. Quoted in Deconstructing Stigma, "Marilyn."
34. Quoted in Brian Krans, "Stigma Still a Major Hurdle in Getting People the Mental Health Care They Need," Healthline, October 20, 2018. www.healthline.com.

Chapter Three: Getting Treatment

35. Joshua David Stein, "Therapy Changed My Life—and I Almost Didn't Do It," Men's Health, May 12, 2020. www.menshealth.com.
36. Stein, "Therapy Changed My Life—and I Almost Didn't Do It."
37. Stein, "Therapy Changed My Life—and I Almost Didn't Do It."
38. Quoted in Alfie Packham and Clea Skopeliti, "'It Gave Me an Ability to Enjoy Life': Readers on Cognitive Behavioural Therapy," *The Guardian* (Manchester, UK), November 4, 2021. www.theguardian.com.
39. Quoted in Packham and Skopeliti, "'It Gave Me an Ability to Enjoy Life.'"
40. Kayla Wright, "How DBT Changed My Life with Borderline Personality Disorder," The Mighty, December 3, 2019. https://themighty.com.

SOURCE NOTES

Introduction: An Everyday Struggle

1. Harry, "Harry's Story: Overcoming Severe Depression," Mental Health Foundation, 2022. www.mentalhealth.org.uk.
2. Harry, "Harry's Story."
3. Harry, "Harry's Story."
4. Harry, "Harry's Story."
5. Quoted in Dave Campbell and Jeff Ayars, "Unmasking Mental Illness and Addiction in a Post-Pandemic World," NBC News, December 18, 2020. www.nbcnews.com.
6. Quoted in US Department of Health and Human Services, "U.S. Surgeon General Issues Advisory on Youth Mental Health Crisis Further Exposed by COVID-19 Pandemic," December 7, 2021. www.hhs.gov.

Chapter One: A View into Mental Illness

7. Nora Super, "Opening Up About My Struggle with Recurring Depression," Health Affairs, 2021. www.healthaffairs.org.
8. Super, "Opening Up About My Struggle with Recurring Depression."
9. Super, "Opening Up About My Struggle with Recurring Depression."
10. Super, "Opening Up About My Struggle with Recurring Depression."
11. Quoted in Rachel Moss, "Five People Who Lost Their Jobs Due to Mental Ill Health Share Their Stories," Huffington Post, October 26, 2017. www.huffingtonpost.co.uk.
12. Quoted in Moss, "Five People Who Lost Their Jobs Due to Mental Ill Health Share Their Stories."
13. Quoted in Moss, "Five People Who Lost Their Jobs Due to Mental Ill Health Share Their Stories."
14. Quoted in Moss, "Five People Who Lost Their Jobs Due to Mental Ill Health Share Their Stories."
15. Quoted in Alina Tugend, "A Climb out of Depression, Doubt and Academic Failure," *New York Times*, June 7, 2017. www.nytimes.com.
16. Quoted in Tugend, "A Climb Out of Depression, Doubt and Academic Failure."

> "My dog helps me navigate my emotional and physical life. . . . I thought nothing could help me, but I'm living life now, even with PTSD and depression."[60]
>
> —Simone, a woman with an emotional support dog to help her manage mental illness

be isolated, but now I see my providers, and I'm outdoors six times a day with my companion dog. I went from walking 20 steps a day to 6,000. My dog helps me navigate my emotional and physical life. . . . I thought nothing could help me, but I'm living life now, even with PTSD and depression."[60]

Overcoming Mental Illness

Mental illness can be a challenging, lifelong condition. However, recovery is possible. With the proper treatment and support, people living with mental illness can find happiness and lead a satisfying life. For many, the first step toward recovery is knowing when to seek help. "The sooner that people take action to get support for their mental health, the more likely it is to be effective,"[61] says Tegan Cruwys, a clinical psychologist and associate professor at the Australian National University.

Nineteen-year-old Finlaey Hewlett has lived with anxiety and depression for almost a decade. She says that seeking help for her mental health and sticking with it changed her life. She says:

> If you don't find a mental health care professional at first who listens to you and understands you, please keep going. It's so easy to be turned off therapy and turned off help when your first experiences are not that pleasant. But keep going because it has honestly changed my life seeking help. It does get better. I know that's so cliche, but recovery isn't a linear process. It's up, and it's down. And it's messy, and it's beautiful. And it's so worth sticking around for.[62]

Spot to Talk

At the Spot to Talk adolescent and children's mental health clinic in Bigfork, Montana, equine therapy helps youth who might need a different approach to treatment. In the program, clients interact with horses while they work with a mental health professional and equine specialist. At Spot to Talk, clients can interact with the horses as much as they want, which gives them the time and space to work through their problems. They do not need to ride, since they can interact with the horses in other ways. Mental health specialist and Spot to Talk owner Claire Wick explains how the therapy works, saying:

> Let's say they want to work on decision-making; I might ask the client to start off with seeing where they can see some decisions being made in the field and we let them just kind of explore. It takes the pressure off of feeling like they have to answer questions and be prepared to talk about something, but really lets them use the space, the props, the equines to find the solution to their story.

Quoted in Taylor Inman, "Spot to Talk Offers Equine Therapy as Mental-Health Resource," *Kalispell (MT) Daily Inter Lake*, November 7, 2021. https://dailyinterlake.com.

Simone, who suffers from PTSD and depression, says that her dog has been a lifeline for her mental health. A few years ago, Simone's mental illness symptoms became debilitating. She could not work and was so anxious and depressed that she did not leave her apartment for six months. Finally, after Simone was hospitalized for her mental health, her psychiatrist recommended that she consider getting an emotional support dog. A few months later, Simone welcomed a dog named Arwen into her home. Since Arwen arrived, Simone's life has improved. "I used to nonriding activity with one of the dozen horses on the farm. Martino might groom a horse or use hand gestures to guide a horse through an obstacle course. "Equine therapy has a positive effect on my mood," says Martino. "I can notice little changes in Indy and then notice them in myself. It has allowed me to start talking about things in my past that would have panicked me before."[59]

Outside of structured therapy, pets provide emotional support and are calming to many people with mental illness. These individuals are often prescribed pets to assist in their well-being. Such pets are referred to as emotional support animals. The most common emotional support animals are dogs and cats, particularly for people with depression. Being around these animals can help reduce stress and anxiety and ease negative feelings. The animals provide reassurance and companionship and help people with mental illness make social connections. Over time, emotional support animals can improve long-term mood and functioning for their owners.

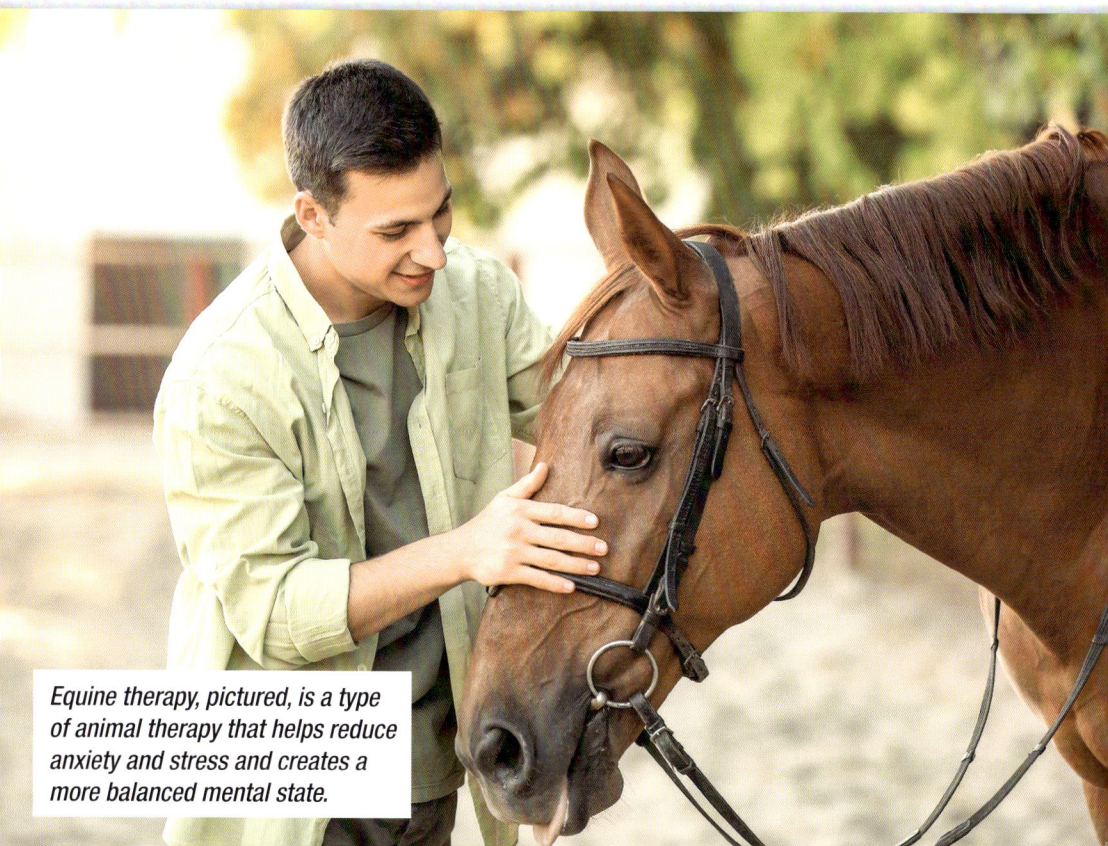

Equine therapy, pictured, is a type of animal therapy that helps reduce anxiety and stress and creates a more balanced mental state.

Animals for Therapy and Emotional Support

Pets and animals provide comfort to people worldwide in many ways. When interacting with a friendly animal, people can form a bond with the animal, producing a calming state for the person. Positive interactions with an animal can help reduce anxiety and stress, reduce feelings of fear and worry, and create a more balanced mental and emotional state.

Sometimes, animals are used as part of a structured therapy program to help people manage and improve mental health. Animal therapy can involve different animals, including dogs, horses, and birds. The animal's handler, who is often its owner, works under the guidance of a doctor to help a person decrease stress and improve mental health. To become an approved therapy animal, the animal and its handler go through several training sessions to become certified. Handlers learn how to interact with people and perform different types of therapies. The animals must pass physical exams to ensure they are healthy and disease-free. Therapy animals also undergo temperament testing to ensure they will behave as expected around people.

Equine therapy is one type of animal therapy that has been helpful for people with depression, anxiety, PTSD, obsessive-compulsive disorder, and substance abuse. At the Bay Meadow Farm, owner and therapist Jen Kraus, a licensed social worker, specializes in equine-assisted therapy. One of her patients is Angela Martino, a twenty-six-year-old Baltimore woman who frequently struggles with anxiety. When Martino lays her hands on the neck of Indy, a gentle, chestnut-colored mare, Martino begins to calm. Her breathing slows and becomes regular. Her shoulders soften, and for the moment, the young woman can focus. "I can't always control where my thoughts go," she says. "But the time I spent with Indy was easy. My anxiety was lower."[58] Most equine therapy sessions begin with Kraus talking with Martino about her feelings. Then Kraus and Martino walk to the barn and start a

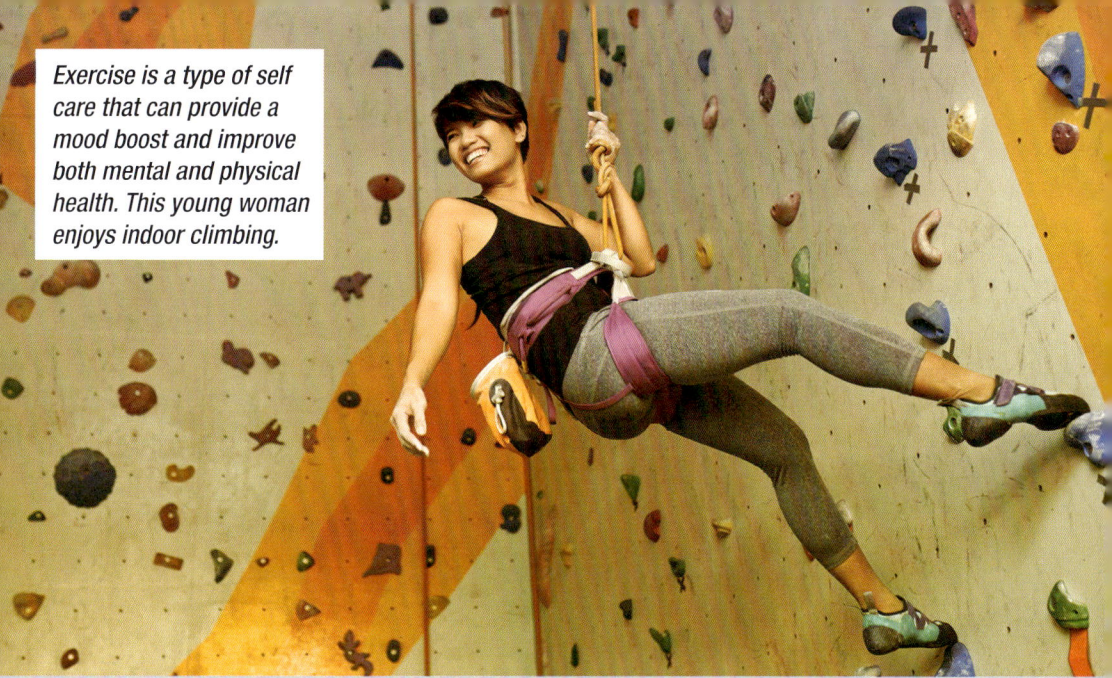

Exercise is a type of self care that can provide a mood boost and improve both mental and physical health. This young woman enjoys indoor climbing.

sense of community and social connections, improving mood and well-being. "People can have a really powerful and transformative experience even if it's not therapy,"[56] says Rachel Brandoff, coordinator of the art therapy specialization in counseling at Thomas Jefferson University.

For Danielle Hark, photography helps manage her depression. The professional writer and photographer stumbled onto this strategy after accidentally snapping a photo of an interesting crack on the wall. She discovered that studying the image shifted her focus quickly away from her depression. "Just that one thought and just that one breath helped me to become more present,"[57] she says. Now Hark uses a variety of creative arts—such as photography, theater, poetry, and mixed-media art—in addition to traditional therapy and medication to help manage her mental health. Every night, she spends hours in a basement studio in an artistic routine that provides structure and purpose. Photography is not a cure for her depression, but it has helped her recovery. When she takes photos, Hark gets out of the house, interacts with people, and transforms things that appear ugly, like cracked sidewalks and crumbling paint, into art. Photography gives Hark a sense of control over her life and mental health.

such as regular exercise and paying close attention to my sleep patterns.[54]

Getting Creative

For some people, getting creative improves mental health. The creative arts—including music, art, dance, theater, writing, photography, and more—relieve stress and promote mental calmness. Creative arts can take one's mind off everyday life and problems and provide a relaxing distraction. Painting gives Jasmine Tot, who lives with depression, a way to control her emotions. When she paints, Tot blends colors, paints in large strokes, and adds details. When she finishes a painting, "I know my emotions are on the canvas, and I can move forward,"[55] she says.

Some people participate in structured creative arts therapy led by a trained therapist. Others pick up a paintbrush, pencil, guitar, or camera themselves. As they express their emotions through painting, movement, film, and more, they can better understand their emotions and find purpose. Some arts programs build a

Learn to Say No

Many people feel overwhelmed when their to-do list grows out of control. They find it hard to say no when asked to take on additional responsibilities, because they want to help or feel bad if they do not. However, taking on too much can become a significant source of stress, which is unhealthy and can impact mental health. Learning to say no in a firm but respectful way does not make one a bad person. It can, however, relieve stress and lead to improved mental health. Saying no can be difficult at first, but when a person's stress levels decline because he or she is not overloaded, it becomes easier to say no in the future.

Yoga may bring additional mental health benefits. The practice of yoga combines stretching and strengthening poses with controlled breathing and meditation. Regular yoga participants claim that it helps them physically and emotionally, strengthening their body and improving mood and emotions. Yoga's mood-elevating effects may occur because it can produce increased levels of gamma-aminobutyric acid, a brain chemical linked to better mood and decreased anxiety. Numerous studies show that yoga can decrease anxiety symptoms, reduce depression, decrease perceived stress, and improve mood. "Yoga seems to have this powerful combination of the physical movement combined with the deep breathing, meditation, and mindfulness aspect," says Dr. Corinna Keenmon, Houston Methodist Hospital's medical director of psychiatry and telepsychiatry. "This total package helps us physically by increasing flexibility, along with heart and brain health. Plus, the cognitive and emotional improvements that happen over time are priceless."[53]

Meditation, as part of yoga or on its own, can also improve mental health. Meditation reduces activity in the brain's limbic system, which controls emotions. Reduced limbic system activity lessens emotional response, which allows a person to have a more moderate response to stressful situations.

Eating well is another self-care strategy to manage mental health. The food people eat affects physical health and can also affect mental health. Eating a balanced diet full of nutrients and vegetables can improve well-being and mood. Diagnosed with schizoaffective disorder, a form of schizophrenia, Will Hall relies on exercise and nutrition to manage his mental health. He says:

> I got off medication and learned about nutrition and changed my diet. I have to avoid milk, caffeine, and sugar, which directly cause my anxiety and symptoms to worsen. . . . I took classes in yoga and meditation and began to see an acupuncturist. . . . I also watch for early warning signs of problems and have wellness tools to support myself,

With his depression under control, Al now talks to mental health providers about the services Face It provides. He says:

> I have been able to talk directly to mental health professionals and tell them just how critical peer support has been in my recovery. . . . What I want other men to know is that recovery IS possible. It's not easy. It takes great effort and consistency and support, but I know firsthand how that effort can pay off. They're not alone in this fight. They shouldn't be afraid to seek out support and talk about their challenges.[51]

Taking Care of Self

Self-care can make living with mental illness easier. Self-care encompasses any act individuals take to improve their physical, mental, and emotional health. Self-care takes many forms. It can include getting enough sleep at night or making sure to get a few minutes of fresh air daily. It can be physical, social, mental, spiritual, or emotional.

Exercise, yoga, and meditation are common forms of self-care that can improve mental health. All forms of exercise boost mood in three ways: lowering stress hormones, increasing the production of feel-good brain chemicals called endorphins, and bringing more oxygenated blood to the brain. As little as thirty minutes of exercise can help boost mood and improve mental and physical health. For Jess, regular rock climbing helps manage her generalized anxiety disorder. "I consider it to be my version of meditation," she says. "All I can think about when I am climbing is climbing. It has been a miracle for my anxiety to be able to completely dump the worries in my head and just think about getting to the top."[52]

> "All I can think about when I am climbing is climbing. It has been a miracle for my anxiety to be able to completely dump the worries in my head and just think about getting to the top."[52]
>
> —Jess, a woman who uses rock climbing to help manage anxiety

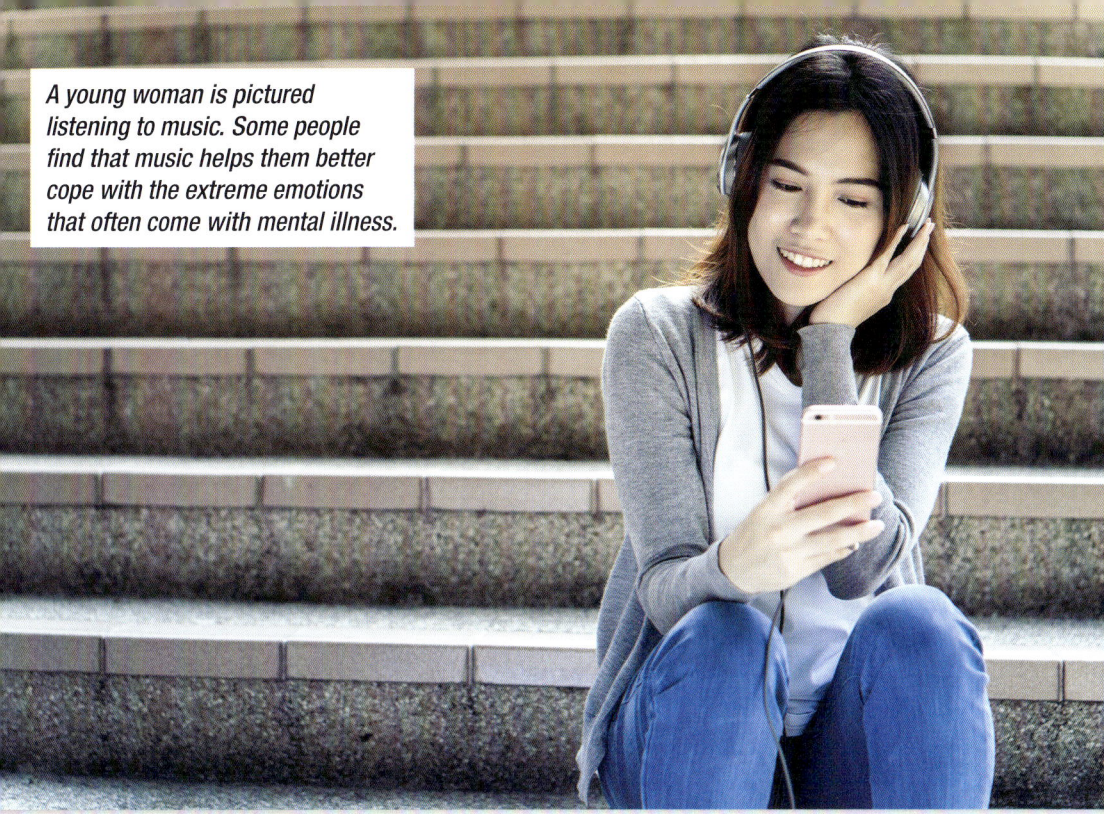

A young woman is pictured listening to music. Some people find that music helps them better cope with the extreme emotions that often come with mental illness.

trouble focusing, and could not get simple tasks done. At home he had no energy for his wife and kids. Sleep was elusive, and he frequently broke down in bouts of sobbing. Then Al began to have detailed thoughts of suicide. He went to see a physician and began taking antidepressant medication. Eventually, Al was admitted into a partial inpatient hospital program. While in the hospital, he attended group therapy sessions to learn how to manage stress.

After being released from the hospital, Al learned about a peer support group for men with depression called Face It. He decided to join one of the Face It groups. He says:

> I'll never forget the first night I walked into the Face It office to attend group. I was scared the guys wouldn't understand my struggles, and I was certain I wouldn't even be able to speak. However, once I had a chance to talk, I think I talked for over an hour. It was the first time I was able to sit down with other men who really understood what I was going through. It was incredibly helpful.[50]

Finding Support on a Lifelong Journey

Living with mental illness is often a lifelong journey. Traditional treatments like psychotherapy and medication can help stabilize individuals in need and teach them skills to manage their mental illness. Many people use additional strategies and self-care practices to help them successfully manage their mental health for a lifetime during and after treatment.

For many people living with mental illness, finding support is essential to long-term recovery. It can be scary to talk about mental health issues with others. However, having a solid support system and trustworthy people to talk to is often essential for recovering and living with mental illness.

Support can come in many forms, including family, friends, teachers, faith leaders, health care providers, and peer support groups. Trusted individuals listen and share while respecting a person's need for confidentiality. They listen to a person's feelings and emotions without judging, teasing, and criticizing and help him or her make a plan for the next time a difficult situation occurs.

In many cases, peer support can be beneficial for overcoming mental illness. Peer support groups bring together people who are also dealing with mental health conditions and have gone through similar experiences. In meetings, group members share stories and coping strategies. Often, peers offer an understanding of how to live with mental illness that others who do not have mental illness cannot provide. They also serve as examples of overcoming mental health problems and living a fulfilling life.

Al, who has depression, says peer support helped him accept and manage his mental illness. For many years Al was reluctant to admit that he had a mental health condition. Then an episode of depression sent him into a tailspin. He struggled at his job, had

> "Whenever I need a moment to myself, I turn my music up loud, pick the best song that will reflect my feelings, and just let it take me."[48]
>
> —Chelsea Hertzog, a woman with depression

CHAPTER FOUR

Lifelong Strategies

For three years, Chelsea Hertzog has been learning to live with depression and generalized anxiety disorder. In addition to traditional mental health treatment, Hertzog has found that music helps her cope with her mental illness. "Music has given my soul hope,"[47] she says.

Hertzog scrolls through songs every day, looking for ones that match her mood. Some days, she listens to a wide range of music genres. When she experiences a depressive episode, Hertzog turns to music to help her manage her emotions. "Whenever I need a moment to myself, I turn my music up loud, pick the best song that will reflect my feelings, and just let it take me. Sometimes during moments of struggle, I don't need [to] make myself feel happy and fake. Instead, I just need to let the pain happen, feel what is real and let the music help me,"[48] she says.

Because of music, Hertzog says she can think more clearly and see things from a different perspective. "I can analyze what I need to do to help myself, and I can start feeling myself again," she says. Hertzog's strategy of using music to help manage her mental illness gives her a way to cope. "I know music will always be a way to escape and help me find peace. When words fail, music speaks,"[49] she says.

al psychotherapy and CBT to group therapy. She found individual therapy to be the most effective for her. She says:

> I do not have a support network of friends and family that I can access, and so I need a professional to listen to me and to let me talk unhindered about my worldview. Outside the therapy room, I tend to put on a front; that everything is fine and I know what I am doing. Within therapy, it is a joy to be allowed to be honest, to be myself, and to know that no matter what I say, I will not be ridiculed but will be treated with kindness and respect.[44]

The relationship between patient and therapist is also critical, according to Malkin. "The challenge of therapy is being honest with yourself and your therapist. It is tempting to hide parts of yourself away and not admit the emotions you are feeling, but you need to be open and to face the things you fear the most. The relationship between you both is the major factor in getting a positive outcome, so you need to have confidence in your therapist,"[45] she says.

Treatment Brings Hope

There is hope with treatment, no matter a person's mental health condition. Many people who get help for their mental illness can manage their symptoms and live happy, productive lives. "The biggest lesson I have learned is to seek out help early. The longer you leave asking for help, the harder it will be to get well again,"[46] says Malkin.

Lack of Access

Every year, millions of Americans struggle to find mental health care when they need it the most. There are several reasons Americans find it difficult to access care. For some people, poor or no insurance coverage and the high cost of treatment are a barrier. According to a 2018 study by Cohen Veterans Network and the National Council for Mental Wellbeing, 25 percent of Americans reported having to choose between paying for necessities and getting mental health treatment. Nearly one in five Americans reported having to choose between treatment for a physical health condition and a mental health condition because of their insurance coverage. For those who can afford mental health treatment, long wait times and limited treatment options are another barrier. According to the same 2018 study, 38 percent of Americans waited more than one week for mental health treatment, while nearly 50 percent have had to (or knew someone who had to) drive more than an hour round trip for treatment.

Treatment Looks Different for Everyone

When dealing with mental health, everyone's treatment plan looks different, and treatments that work for one person may not work for another person. Even for people with the same diagnosis, mental illness and its symptoms can appear differently. Therefore, the most effective mental health treatment is the one that is specifically tailored for an individual patient.

Vicky Malkin knows firsthand how it can take time to find the mental health treatment that works. The fifty-eight-year-old administrative assistant from Greater Manchester, England, first went to therapy for her depression at age seventeen. Over the years, she participated in different types of therapy, from individu-

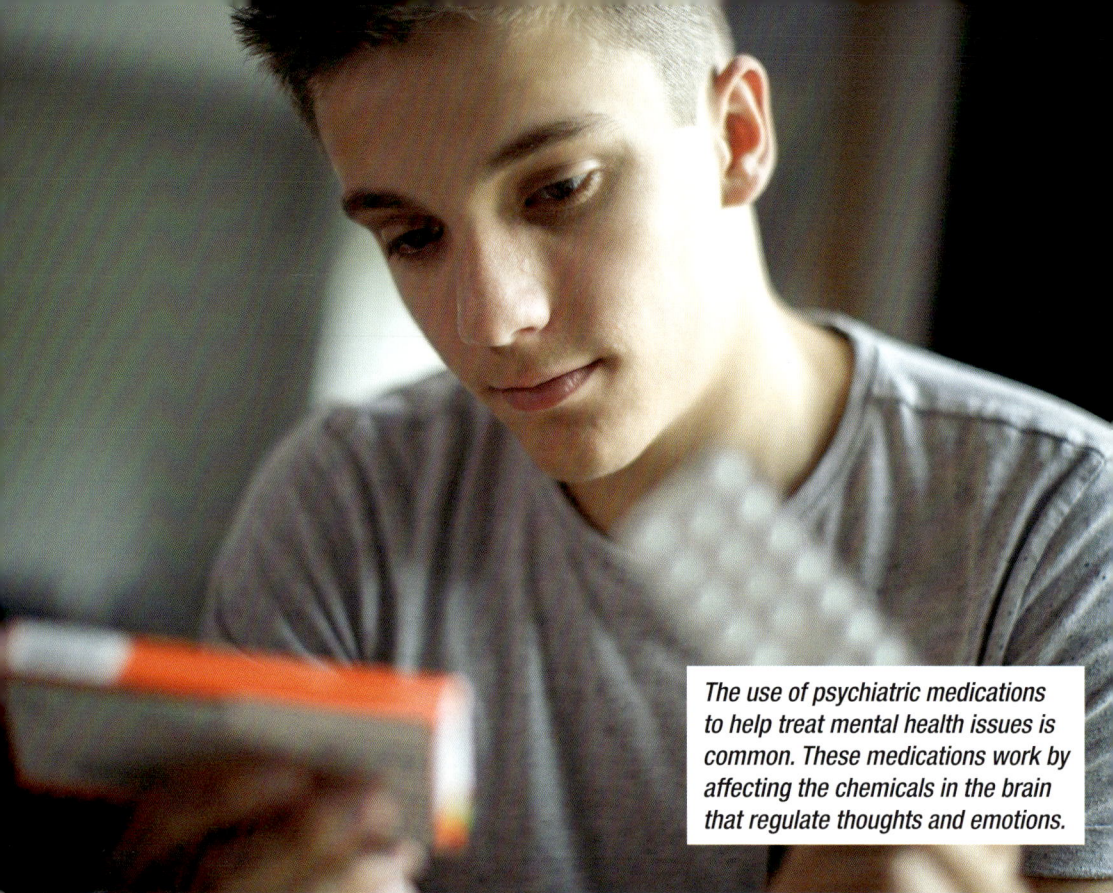

The use of psychiatric medications to help treat mental health issues is common. These medications work by affecting the chemicals in the brain that regulate thoughts and emotions.

For Lily Burana, finding the right combination of medications has been a trial-and-error process. Burana lives with three mental health issues: anxiety, depression, and attention-deficit/hyperactivity disorder. A combination of medication and therapy has helped her overcome these conditions and live her life. "Finding the proper medication, or medications, to treat overlapping mental health conditions is more often a wavy course than a straight line, as exhibited by my own trial-and-error," she says. "With vigilance, plus medication and regular therapy, I feel mostly OK, most of the time. My work gets done, my obligations met; the black-dog days stand stark in their rare awfulness,"[43] she says.

> "Finding the proper medication, or medications, to treat overlapping mental health conditions is more often a wavy course than a straight line."[43]
>
> —Lily Burana, a woman with anxiety, depression, and attention-deficit/hyperactivity disorder

relationships with others and aims to improve the patient's interpersonal skills.

Medication

For many people, mental health treatment includes medication. Psychiatric medications work by affecting the brain chemicals that regulate thoughts and emotions. In some cases mental health medications reduce symptoms to make other treatments such as therapy more effective. For example, for a patient with depression, medication can ease symptoms such as low energy and difficulty concentrating. Reducing these symptoms allows the patient to participate more fully in psychotherapy.

Mental health medications fall into several main categories. Antipsychotic medications are typically used to treat schizophrenia, mania, bipolar disorder, and treatment-resistant depression. These drugs reduce or eliminate the delusions and hallucinations common in these conditions by acting on the brain chemical dopamine. Antidepressants improve depression symptoms by affecting serotonin, norepinephrine, and dopamine, the brain chemicals linked to emotion. Antianxiety medications reduce the physical and emotional symptoms of anxiety. They are often prescribed to treat phobias, generalized anxiety disorder, and panic disorder. Mood stabilizers treat the mood swings associated with bipolar disorder. In some cases mental health medications are used short term and are only needed for a few months. Other medications are used long term and may become part of a person's lifelong treatment plan.

Finding the proper medication or combination of medications can take time. Some medications work quickly, but others work more slowly and take weeks to months to be fully effective. Some mental health medications also cause side effects. If patients feel as if a medication is not working or is causing unpleasant side effects, they should talk to their doctor about adjusting the medication or dosage.

less pain. At that point the therapist will help the patient replace the negative emotions with healthier thoughts and associations.

David Barge spent many years in therapy to deal with the pain, grief, depression, and anger caused by past traumas in his life. One therapist suggested that he try EMDR. He says:

> I had experienced many things that had left me scarred and stuck. Normal adult experiences could easily and unhelpfully take me back into earlier troubling experiences (those which made me feel deeply upset and sick when I recalled them). So levels of anxiety, fear, anger, and depression could be triggered by events *now* which I knew were way out of proportion to what was actually happening.[41]

After several EMDR sessions, Barge could sense a positive shift in his mental health. Five years later, Barge's traumatic memories no longer produce deep feelings. "They are where they belong. Neutralized and in the past. Yes, they happened—but that was THEN, not NOW," he says. "I'm now sixty-two—and can say with some confidence that the burdens which have plagued me all my life have been laid to rest. I no longer experience depression or inappropriate anger. I feel strong, empowered, and alive. I am fortunate. EMDR transformed my life."[42]

> "I no longer experience depression or inappropriate anger. I feel strong, empowered, and alive. I am fortunate. EMDR transformed my life."[42]
>
> —David Barge, a man with depression and PTSD

Other forms of psychotherapy include exposure therapy and interpersonal therapy. Exposure therapy is a form of CBT frequently used to treat patients with obsessive-compulsive disorder, PTSD, and various phobias. Patients are exposed in a controlled way to the situations and objects that trigger anxiety or ritual behaviors, and they practice using coping strategies to lessen anxiety or stop performing rituals. Interpersonal therapy focuses on a patient's of dealing with it. DBT taught me how to feel my emotions in a healthy way, how to feel an emotion without giving it power to take over. I learned emotions have a purpose, and we can learn a lot from them.[40]

Reducing Stress from Past Traumas

Another type of psychotherapy, eye movement desensitization and reprocessing (EMDR) therapy, can help patients with post-traumatic stress disorder (PTSD) reduce the emotional distress caused by past traumas. Under a therapist's guidance, a patient moves his or her eyes back and forth, left to right, while thinking about a trauma that causes great discomfort. This movement mimics the eye movement during specific periods of sleep when memories are reprocessed and stored. In EMDR this eye movement while thinking about trauma helps the brain reprocess the traumatic memories. Over several sessions the emotions connected to these memories often become less intense and cause

Hospitalization

Sometimes, mental illness becomes so severe that a person needs to be hospitalized. Hospitalization is often voluntary, but it can be involuntary if individuals are believed to be a threat to themselves or others. People may benefit from hospitalization if they are having severe mental health symptoms, hallucinations, delusions, or suicidal or homicidal thoughts; are unable to eat or sleep for days; or are unable to care for themselves because of mental health symptoms. In the hospital, health care providers closely monitor patients; administer medication, fluids, and nutrition; and provide other emergency care. The goal of hospitalization is to stabilize patients so that they are able to move forward with longer-term treatment.

which she openly explored her behaviors, triggers, and feelings. Although she still struggles with her mental health condition, Jasmine now sees hope for the future. "My trichotillomania might take years to dissipate—if at all—but my ability to cope with it has dramatically improved. The iceberg is big but, thanks to CBT, it finally seems surmountable,"[39] she says.

Taking Control of Uncomfortable Thoughts

For others, dialectical behavioral therapy (DBT) has proved successful at treating mental illness. DBT is often used to treat people with borderline personality disorder but can be used for other mental health conditions. DBT is similar to CBT; however, it stresses accepting uncomfortable thoughts, feelings, and behaviors. The therapist helps the patient find a balance between acceptance and finding a way to change. The therapist works with the patient to learn new skills, coping methods, and mindfulness practices to change and improve unhealthy thoughts and behaviors. Improving a patient's coping skills is an essential part of successful treatment.

For Kayla Wright, DBT helped her cope with borderline personality disorder. Before DBT, Wright was consumed by obsessive, intrusive thoughts. She pushed away family and friends and struggled with self-harm tendencies. To get help, she entered a ten-month inpatient DBT program. It changed her life. Wright says:

> I used to be ruled by obsessive, intrusive thoughts so badly it was as though they were personas that took over at different times. I still have intrusive thoughts, but I've learned thoughts aren't facts, they only have the power we give them. I control my thoughts. And I'll tell you now, that wasn't a fast or easy thing to learn. It took time and practice, but it was more than worth the effort it took. I used to lash out at my family, over really small things because I'd let my anger build up and I'd just push it down instead

health conditions, including depression, anxiety disorders, bipolar disorder, eating disorders, and schizophrenia.

For twenty-one-year-old Jasmine from Bracknell, England, CBT has dramatically improved her ability to cope with mental illness. Jasmine suffers from trichotillomania, a compulsive hair-pulling disorder. Since age thirteen, Jasmine has been pulling out the hairs on her legs and hands, leaving scabs across her body. "It can seem like a trivial issue, but it has impacted almost every facet of my life. I lose track of time once I've started a pulling episode; my sense of self and body image is completely [ruined]. I've lost sleep and skipped meals because of it,"[38] she says.

At age sixteen, Jasmine sought help from a counselor who tried to help her develop creative distraction techniques when she felt the urge to pull hairs. When she started college, Jasmine struggled to cope, and her pulling episodes began to disrupt her work. She reached out to the university counseling service for help. Working with university counselors, she started CBT, in

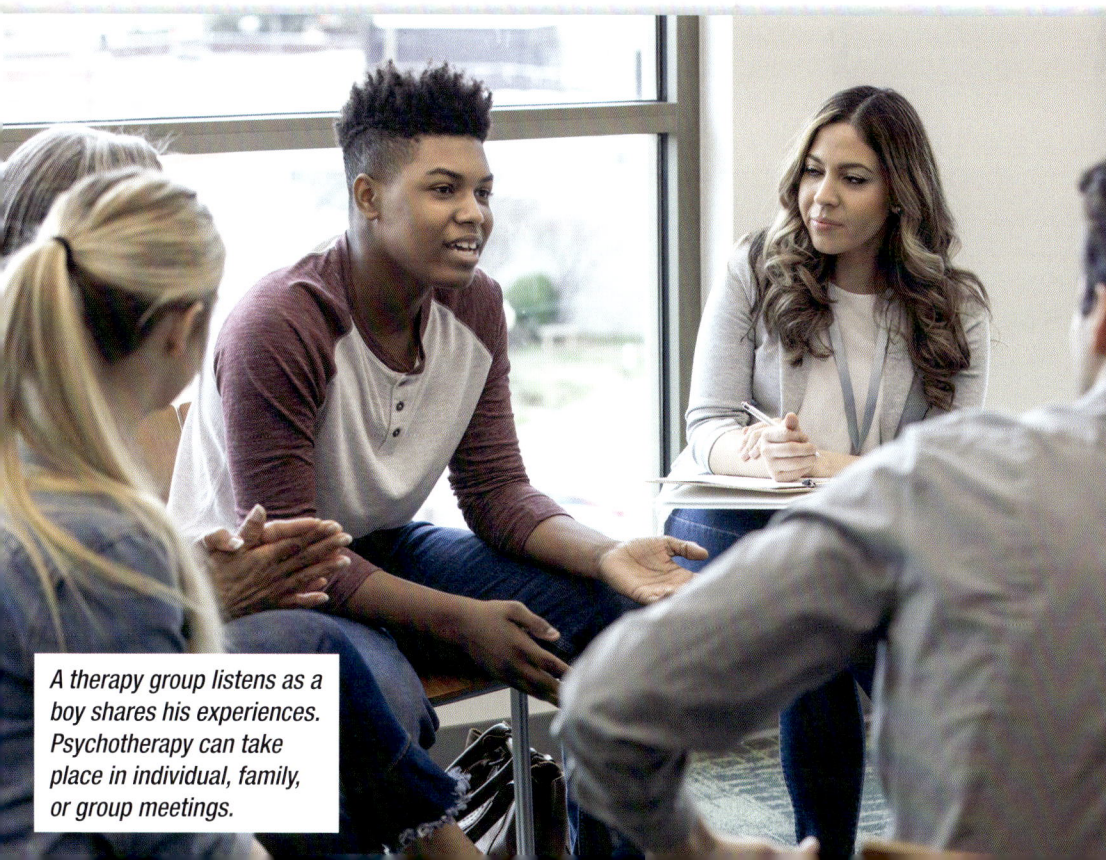

A therapy group listens as a boy shares his experiences. Psychotherapy can take place in individual, family, or group meetings.

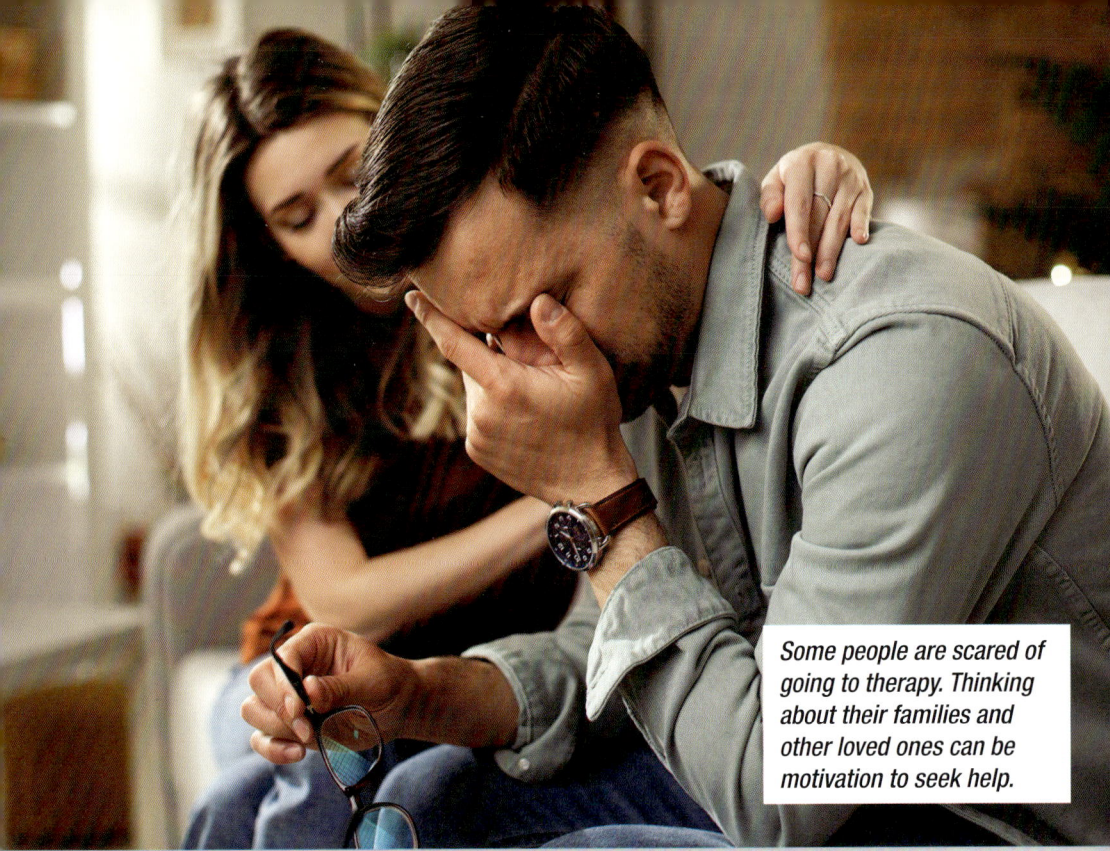

Some people are scared of going to therapy. Thinking about their families and other loved ones can be motivation to seek help.

known as talk therapy, patients talk with a trained therapist in a safe and confidential setting. Psychotherapy can occur in individual, group, or family meetings. In a therapy session, the therapist and patient discuss past and current problems, experiences, thoughts, and feelings. Patients explore their feelings and learn to understand their triggers and behaviors. They practice skills to cope with their mental illness.

One of the most common types of psychotherapy used for mental illness is cognitive behavioral therapy (CBT). In CBT, a therapist works with a patient to help him or her recognize unhealthy patterns of thoughts and see how these may be causing unhealthy behaviors, feelings, and beliefs. By identifying these patterns, the patient and therapist can work together to learn new ways of thinking, resulting in healthier behaviors and thoughts. For example, CBT can help a patient recognize thoughts that lead to low self-esteem and replace them with positive thoughts. Studies have shown that CBT effectively treats many mental

There are many reasons people do not seek treatment for mental health conditions. For some, the stigma and shame of admitting to mental illness and receiving treatment prevent them from asking for help. For others, poverty and lack of insurance to pay for treatment act as barriers. Some people have trouble finding a therapist they trust, and others do not like the side effects that medications for depression, anxiety, and other mental illnesses can cause. Also, mental illness can be isolating and disruptive to daily life, making it more challenging to find the proper treatment. As a result, many people continue to struggle without treatment for their condition.

Mental health conditions rarely get better without help, and the longer the illness lasts, the harder it can be to treat and recover. Untreated, mental health symptoms often worsen. For example, untreated anxiety can intensify and trigger panic attacks. In addition, untreated mental illness can also cause physical problems. Over time, people may experience aches, pains, and gastrointestinal problems with no apparent physical cause. The stress of chronic mental illness can also increase the risk of stroke, heart disease, and obesity.

Untreated mental illness can also lead to instability in daily life, making it hard to keep a job or maintain relationships. And in some cases, untreated mental illness can become so severe that a person thinks about ending his or her life. According to the NAMI, research has found that 46 percent of people who commit suicide have a known mental health condition.

Psychotherapy: Talk-Based Treatment

Effective treatment is different for every person and every mental health condition. Treatment can take place in various settings and involve a team of providers such as psychologists, psychiatrists, counselors, nurses, and peer support professionals.

For many people, psychotherapy is one of the most effective treatments for mental health conditions. In psychotherapy, also someone who wasn't furious at me for a decade of craziness, who could see me with compassion and professional compunction,"[36] he says. After several sessions, Julia suggested that Stein might have borderline personality disorder, which causes symptoms such as suicidal thoughts, uncontrollable rage, impulsive behavior, and black-and-white thinking. Stein immediately recognized himself in the description of the mental health condition. The more he learned about the illness, the more he understood what he had been feeling.

Today Stein credits mental health therapy with helping him learn how to manage his mental health and live his best life. While it was not enough to save his marriage, therapy did help Stein understand himself better. He says:

> It's like I hadn't fully put my weight on this earth. I was holding part of myself apart, suspended, like a terrified marionette. Now I'm here. I'm happy in a way I couldn't be before and sad in a way I couldn't be before. I'm tender where I was hard, looser where I was tight. And you know what? I'm more comfortable admitting, "I'm scared," and still going to sit on a couch to get to know myself a little better.[37]

Missing Out on Treatment

As Stein's story illustrates, seeking help for mental health conditions is an essential part of coping with and overcoming mental illness. However, according to Mental Health America, more than half of American adults with a mental health condition do not receive treatment. Many American youths are also going without mental health treatment. For example, more than 60 percent of youth with major depression do not receive any mental health treatment. According to Mental Health America, for those with severe depression who are receiving some care, less than one in three youth are getting consistent treatment.

CHAPTER THREE

Getting Treatment

As a young, married father, Joshua David Stein's life was falling apart. His marriage was in turmoil, and his emotions were out of control. He struggled with intense rage and severe sadness. Feeling miserable had long been a part of his identity, so he had never sought professional help for his mental health struggles. In 2018 Stein's mental health deteriorated to the point that he experienced a mental breakdown and tried to commit suicide.

However, thinking about his young children stopped Stein from killing himself. He says:

> At that point, seeking help was a matter of life and death for me. Even then, I dithered out of fear. But what scared me more than going to therapy was what not going would mean. The evidence that I was struggling with mental illness was incontrovertible; that it was affecting the people I love was equally uncontestable. Because I have children and love my children, I knew I needed to get help, not for me so much as for them.[35]

Stein began therapy with a counselor named Julia. At first, he was skeptical that their weekly sessions would help him. "But week by week, it felt really good to be able to talk to

This Is My Brave

Nationwide, several organizations and campaigns aim to reduce mental health stigma and discrimination. One example, This Is My Brave, is a storytelling theater show in which people share their stories of how they are able to live successfully with mental illness. Since its first show in 2014, This Is My Brave has produced more than 75 shows across the United States that highlight the stories of nearly 875 individuals. In the shows, the storytellers detail their real-life experiences overcoming depression, anxiety, post-traumatic stress disorder, bipolar disorder, and other mental illnesses. In 2017 This Is My Brave expanded beyond the United States into Australia. "Our message is we want to reduce the stigma by putting names and faces to their true stories of recovery so they know mental illness and addiction can happen to anyone. But there is hope and they can find ways to live through it," says This Is My Brave's executive director, Erin Gallagher.

Quoted in Karen Graham, "Ashburn-based nonprofit 'This Is My Brave' Announces New Leadership," *Loudoun Times-Mirror*, December 1, 2021. www.loudountimes.com.

Do Not Delay—Get Help

Stigma can cause people to feel ashamed of their mental health. Even worse, stigma can prevent people from getting the help they need. Delaying or avoiding mental health treatment can worsen symptoms and make a recovery more difficult.

According to Natasha Tracy, a mental health writer who has bipolar disorder, the most challenging stigma to overcome is the one that "looks back at us in the mirror." It can take years to stop feeling bad about their mental health problems for some people. And like any physical illness, mental illness will not go away without treatment. Tracy urges people to stop worrying about others' thoughts and instead focus on themselves and get better. "It can be difficult if people around you can't accept your mental illness treatment, but first and foremost, treatment is about getting you better,"[34] says Tracy.

Marilyn almost let mental health stigma stop her from seeking treatment. Growing up, she had always had some symptoms of anxiety. As an adult, her symptoms worsened, and she experienced severe panic attacks. One night while she was watching television, an infomercial talked about panic disorder. Marilyn says:

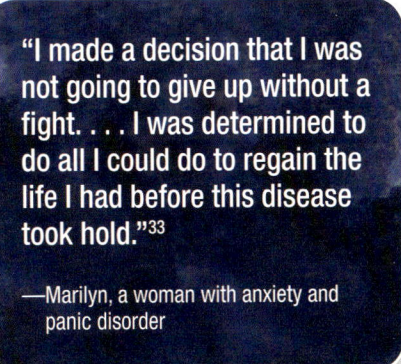

"I made a decision that I was not going to give up without a fight. . . . I was determined to do all I could do to regain the life I had before this disease took hold."[33]

—Marilyn, a woman with anxiety and panic disorder

> The host described everything that I was experiencing, and I sat up in bed recognizing that they were describing me! . . . I then had to make a hard decision on what I was going to do about it. At the time of my introductory journey into the darkness of mental illness, there was a great deal of stigma attached to these conditions. The thought that I needed to seek psychiatric help was unnerving. It caused me great concern knowing that people would perceive me differently if they knew I had to seek psychiatric help.[32]

However, Marilyn ultimately decided to get help. With medication and therapy, she regained control of her life. She says:

> I remember when I had to take a 30-day leave of absence from work due to my illness. . . . At that point in my life, I was feeling like such a failure. The disease was winning. But I made a decision that I was not going to give up without a fight. I made up my mind that in no way [was] this how I was going to spend the rest of my life. I was determined to do all I could do to regain the life I had before this disease took hold.[33]

Today Marilyn encourages other people who fear the stigma of mental illness to fight this fear and move forward with recovery.

Sometimes the stigma of mental illness starts within oneself. Some people with mental illness believe their symptoms are simply a sign of personal weakness, and they think they should be able to "tough it out" or "get over it" without asking for help. However, learning about mental illness and talking to others who have similar conditions can help people reduce self-stigma and allow them to seek help. "I fight stigma by not having stigma for myself—not hiding from this world in shame, but being a productive member of society," says Jamie Brown, who lives with mental illness. "I volunteer at church, have friends, and I'm a peer mentor and a mom. I take my treatment seriously. I'm purpose driven and want to show others they can live a meaningful life even while battling [mental illness]."[30]

Stigma can also cause people to hide their symptoms. However, friends and family cannot help if they are kept in the dark. Reaching out to trusted friends, family, and advisers can help individuals get the support they need. Sometimes, people with mental illness find understanding in support groups with others who have similar experiences. Rather than hiding their conditions, some people actively try to share their stories and educate others about mental illness. Sara Bean, who lives with mental illness, says:

> "I fight stigma by not having stigma for myself—not hiding from this world in shame, but being a productive member of society."[30]
>
> —Jamie Brown, a woman with mental illness

> I take every opportunity to educate people and share my personal story and struggles with mental illness. It doesn't matter where I am, if I overhear a conversation or a rude remark being made about mental illness, or anything regarding a similar subject, I always try to use that as a learning opportunity and gently intervene and kindly express how this makes me feel, and how we need to stop this because it only adds to the stigma.[31]

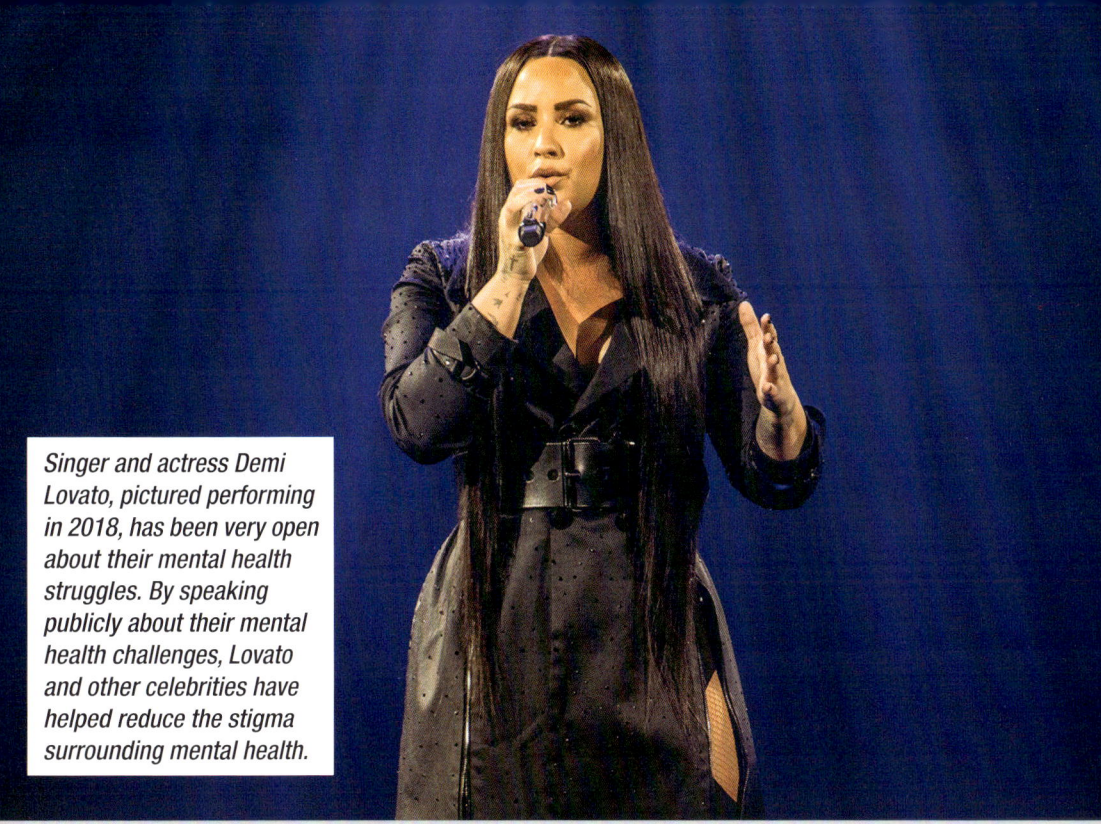

Singer and actress Demi Lovato, pictured performing in 2018, has been very open about their mental health struggles. By speaking publicly about their mental health challenges, Lovato and other celebrities have helped reduce the stigma surrounding mental health.

Lovato does more than talk about mental illness. The singer has also organized wellness workshops with a personal-development coach before most shows to discuss mental health issues with fans. At one such workshop, Lovato walked in with manager Phil McIntyre and singers Joe and Nick Jonas. Joe Jonas and McIntyre spoke to the crowd about their mental health challenges. When others see these successful people talk openly about their mental health struggles, it helps reduce the shame that often comes with these feelings.

Coping with the Stigma of Mental Illness

People who are struggling with mental illness may be reluctant to admit they have a problem and need treatment. However, the fear of being labeled as having a mental illness should not prevent them from getting the help they need. Treatment can pinpoint what is wrong and help people reduce the symptoms that impact their daily lives.

Stigma in the Workplace

Mental health stigma remains a significant issue at work. While many employers offer employee assistance programs that provide mental health services, employees are often reluctant to take advantage of these programs because of stigma. In a 2019 nationwide poll from the American Psychiatric Association, about 50 percent of employees responded that they were concerned about talking about mental health at work. More than one in three said they worried about retaliation or being fired if they sought mental health treatment. However, there may be some hope that attitudes are changing. The poll found that younger workers were almost twice as likely as older workers to be comfortable talking about their mental health at work.

Many celebrities have also talked publicly about their mental health challenges. Celebrities such as Demi Lovato, Michael Phelps, Lady Gaga, and Dwayne Johnson have shared their mental health stories with the world. By being open about their mental health, they have helped make it easier to talk about and reduce the stigma surrounding mental health.

Singer and actress Demi Lovato has been very open about mental health struggles. The singer was diagnosed with bipolar disorder in 2010 after a lifelong battle with mental illness. Since entering treatment, Lovato has become an advocate for people to come out about their mental health. "Like millions of Americans, I am living with mental illness," Lovato said before a performance in 2016. "But I am lucky. I had the resources and support to get treatment at a top facility. Unfortunately, too many Americans from all walks of life don't get help, whether they fear the stigma or cannot afford treatment."[29]

don't talk about mental illness. You suck it up and deal with it,"[27] she says. Dominque could no longer ignore her mental health in college and went to a doctor for help. She was diagnosed with anxiety and depression and began treatment. Dominique hopes others will learn from her experiences. She wants people in the Black community to speak up about mental health and realize that it is okay to ask for help. "The hardest part of fixing a problem is acknowledging its existence. We have to stop making it seem like it's not okay to not be okay," she says. Ignoring mental health will only make things worse, she insists. "Not only does it invalidate the reality of these issues within our community, but it also reinforces unhealthy coping mechanisms."[28]

Reducing the Stigma of Mental Illness

The stigma of mental illness is often rooted in fear of the unknown. Research shows that when people know someone with mental illness, they are more likely to understand mental health. Knowing someone dealing with mental health problems can make it less scary and more real.

When people with mental illness speak out and share their stories, it puts a human face on the illness and can help reduce stigma. For young people in particular, learning about others' mental health struggles can make these conditions less scary and encourage these youths to seek help for their problems. Often, young people turn to the internet to learn about mental health and connect with others' personal stories. In 2020 a survey of fourteen- to twenty-two-year-olds in the United States found that 90 percent of teens and young adults who experienced depression symptoms turned to online sources to research mental health issues. Also, 75 percent used the internet to access personal mental health stories via blogs, podcasts, and online videos.

> "The hardest part of fixing a problem is acknowledging its existence. We have to stop making it seem like it's not okay to not be okay."[28]
>
> —Dominque, a woman with anxiety and depression

shame to a family. These cultural beliefs can make it difficult for people to talk about their mental health and ask for help.

Ramya is part of a South Asian culture, which she admits prevented her from seeking help for mental health. Growing up, she often heard words like *weak* and *crazy* when people talked about others with mental health conditions. As a result, Ramya tried to dismiss her mental health symptoms, which proved to be damaging. "I didn't get help or even acknowledge what was going on with me,"[24] she says.

Only when Ramya moved far away from her hometown could she get help. In a new place, she could talk about her mental health, feelings, and past traumas without the fear of someone she knew finding out. In talk therapy, Ramya learned strategies and coping mechanisms to deal with her mental health. Even more importantly, she no longer felt ashamed of her condition. "I could be the role model and the girl with a mental illness," she says. "It wasn't a reason to be made fun of or be told to 'suck it up.' I didn't need to call myself names anymore. I felt for the first time that I was going to be okay."[25]

Today Ramya wishes she had ignored the stigma and gotten help for her mental health earlier. A graduate of Columbia University, she works as a social worker and advocates for mental health. "I want to live in a world where people don't stop themselves from getting better because of stigma, and I will do everything I can to fight that for the people who come after me,"[26] she says.

> "I want to live in a world where people don't stop themselves from getting better because of stigma."[26]
>
> —Ramya, a social worker who lives with mental illness

A member of the Black community, Dominique has experienced the stigma of mental illness herself. Starting when she was twelve years old, she began experiencing anxiety. By her senior year of high school, Dominique had panic attacks daily. Even though her mental health significantly impacted her daily life, she did not tell anyone about her struggles. "In my community, we

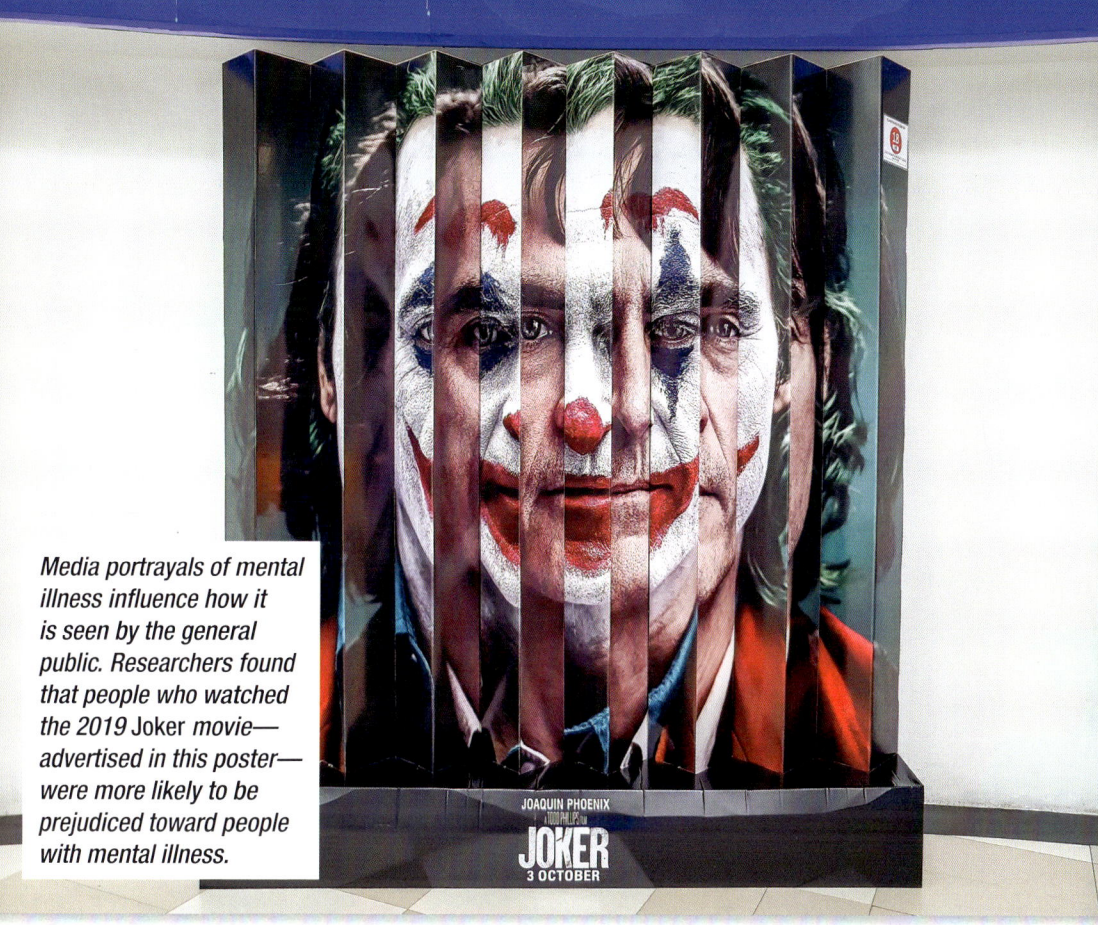

Media portrayals of mental illness influence how it is seen by the general public. Researchers found that people who watched the 2019 Joker movie—advertised in this poster—were more likely to be prejudiced toward people with mental illness.

feeling sad" when they have not experienced mental health problems themselves. Also, misunderstanding of mental illness is often made worse by misleading portrayals of mental illness in the media. In a study published in 2020, researchers examined the effect of the 2019 movie *Joker* on how people saw mental illness. The lead character has a mental illness in the movie and becomes extremely violent. Researchers found that people who watched the film were more likely to have higher levels of prejudice toward people with mental illness than those who did not watch the movie.

Growing Up with Stigma

Every culture views mental health differently. In many cultures, there is a stigma around mental health, and mental health problems are viewed as a weakness and something to hide. In some cultures, seeking mental health treatment is viewed as bringing

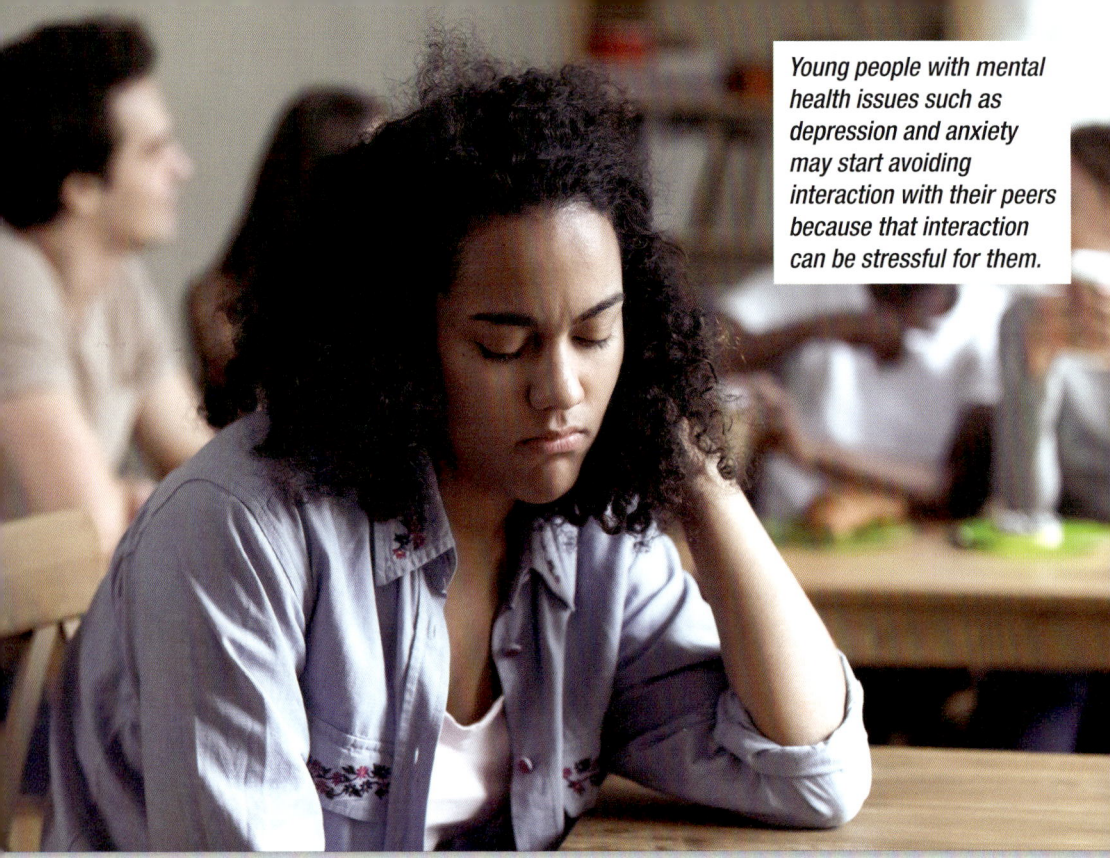

Young people with mental health issues such as depression and anxiety may start avoiding interaction with their peers because that interaction can be stressful for them.

than half of people with mental illness do not receive help for their conditions. Often, people may not seek treatment or may delay needed treatment because they are afraid of what others will think about them or are ashamed to admit they have a problem. Many people fear that admitting to mental illness will cause others to treat them differently or even cost them their job.

Stigma occurs when someone views another person negatively because of a specific characteristic or personal trait. Stigma can lead to prejudice and discrimination. Sometimes, discrimination can be direct, such as when someone makes a negative comment about a person's mental illness or treatment. Other times, discrimination can be more subtle, perhaps avoiding others who might be mentally ill because of an assumption that they could be unstable or violent.

Fear and stigma surrounding mental illness often occur because people do not understand mental illness. It may be difficult for others to understand why someone cannot just "snap out of it" or "stop even get out of bed in the morning to go to class. I felt paralyzed when I woke up," he says. To escape, Vic turned to binge drinking alcohol. "While the alcohol helped in the moment, I always felt worse off afterwards,"[22] he says. Feeling hopeless, Vic thought about suicide.

For years Vic's negative experiences talking to family and friends about his mental health had stopped him from seeking help. Now he decided to visit the counseling center at his university. He says:

> I remember my first appointment vividly. I had walked in and burst into tears about how I felt. The counselor was very understanding, and I learned that I had Generalized Anxiety Disorder or GAD. I continued to seek counseling services after this appointment and began opening up to some of my classmates about how I felt. To my surprise, some of them had felt this way too and were very open with me talking about this.[23]

Vic finally found the support he needed at the counseling center to talk through his feelings and learned healthy ways to channel his emotions. He started to exercise regularly and ate better. He also started taking antianxiety medications. Volunteering with local nonprofit organizations helped give him a sense of purpose. While Vic still experiences anxiety today, he has learned how to deal with his mental health through treatment and counseling so that it no longer derails his daily life.

Fear and Stigma

For most people the first step in facing mental illness is recognizing the condition and knowing when to seek help. However, as Vic experienced, the stigma of mental illness and other barriers to treatment often prevent people from getting help when they need it. According to the American Psychiatric Association, more

CHAPTER TWO

Overcoming the Stigma of Mental Illness

When Vic started high school, he began to feel increasingly anxious. His class schedule overwhelmed him, and he struggled to keep up with his classmates. Unhappy, he started having trouble sleeping at night. And he began to hide in the bathroom during class to avoid contact with peers and teachers.

When Vic tried to talk to his family and friends about his anxiety at school, they told him to calm down and dismissed his feelings. One family member accused Vic of making up his mental health troubles to get extra attention. "This was very hard on me," Vic says. "I began to refrain from telling people how I felt. This only made me feel worse about myself. I started to feel very depressed. While I felt this way, I put on a facade like nothing was wrong."[21]

In college, Vic's mental health problems worsened. His anxiety made him too nervous to interact with other students, making it difficult to make new friends. To escape, Vic walked around campus with his head and eyes down so he would not have to make eye contact. Other times, he hid alone in his dorm room. Vic's depression and anxiety increasingly began to impact his daily life. "There would be points where I didn't it was something people did. I remember crying a lot and thinking, Why did I just do that? I was kind of scared of myself,"[20] she says. However, the cutting made some of her anxiety dissipate. To get relief from her feelings, Joan began to cut regularly, with knives and then razor blades. She cut her wrists and forearms and moved on to most of her body. Now sixteen, Joan is working to reduce her cutting and manage her mental health in a healthier way.

At some point in their lives, everyone experiences feelings of fear, worry, sadness, and distress. These feelings do not last long and do not affect daily life for most people. However, for some people these feelings can become intense and develop into a mental health disorder that disrupts their ability to function in normal daily activities. Early recognition and treatment improve the likelihood of a successful recovery for people with mental health disorders.

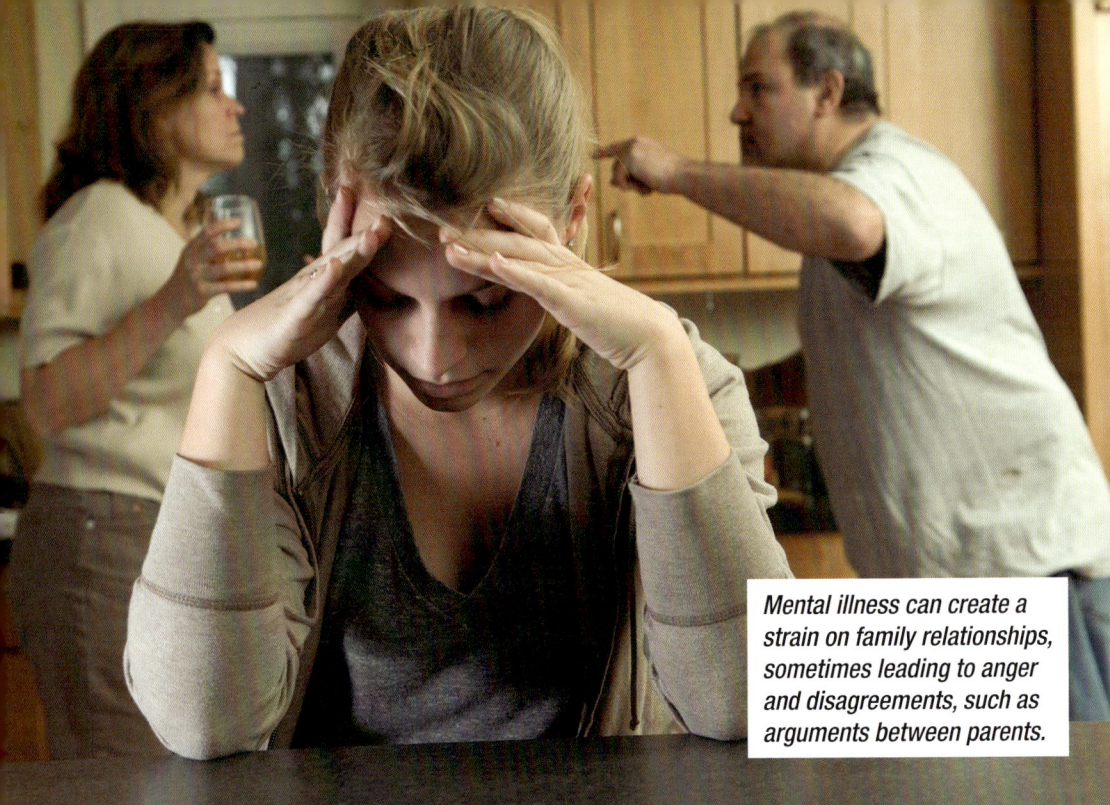

Mental illness can create a strain on family relationships, sometimes leading to anger and disagreements, such as arguments between parents.

pleasure. Other times, people may self-harm to make themselves feel pain instead of feeling emotionally numb. "You cut for different reasons," says sixteen-year-old Blue, a high school student who cuts herself. "Like, it's the only way you know to deal with intense insecurities or anger at yourself. Or you're so numb as a result of depression, you can't feel anything—and this is one thing you can feel."[19] Self-harm behaviors can trigger feelings of guilt and shame, prompting other self-harm behaviors and starting a dangerous cycle.

New York City high school student Joan knows all too well how mental illness can drive a person to self-harm. Overwhelmed by sadness, anxiety, and shame, Joan started cutting when she was thirteen. "I had this Popsicle stick and carved it into a sharp point and scratched myself. I'm not even sure where the idea came from. I just knew

> "You cut for different reasons. Like, it's the only way you know to deal with intense insecurities or anger at yourself. Or you're so numb as a result of depression, you can't feel anything—and this is one thing you can feel."[19]
>
> —Blue, a student with mental illness

calls or conversations, continued concerns over their loved one's health and wellbeing, and overhanging fear of a potential suicide attempt. When pressed, fatigued, and frustrated, family members may snap out hurtful or counterproductive comments. That leads to further anger and resentment.[18]

Risky Behaviors

Sometimes, mental illness can lead to risky behaviors. At times, people may turn to alcohol or drugs to self-medicate and relieve depression, anxiety, and other mental illnesses. However, the effect of these substances is often temporary. Instead of providing lasting relief, alcohol and drugs may make mental health symptoms worse over time. And the longer individuals use addictive drugs and alcohol, the higher their risk of developing a substance abuse disorder.

> "Dealing with a family member who has a mood disorder or anxiety can require a lot of effort from a family member—at times, it can even be exhausting."[18]
>
> —Dr. Susan Noonan, a mental health peer specialist

In some cases, people with mental illness can become a threat to harm themselves or others. Some people feel the urge to burn themselves, pull out hair, pick at wounds, or cut themselves with a sharp object. Regardless of the method, hurting oneself or thinking about it is a sign of emotional and mental distress. While self-harm is not a mental illness, it is often a sign of underlying mental illness such as depression, eating disorders, anxiety, or post-traumatic stress disorder.

Self-harm behaviors most often occur in teens and young adults. The urge to hurt oneself may begin with feelings of anger, frustration, or pain. When a person cannot deal with these uncomfortable emotions, self-harm behaviors can become a way to escape. Sometimes, self-harm stimulates the body to release endorphins, which are hormones that reduce pain and increase

Warning Signs

There is no easy test to determine whether a person has a mental illness. However, there are several warning signs and symptoms that may indicate a person may have a mental health problem. These can include excessive worry or fear, excessive sadness, confusion, difficulty concentrating, extreme mood changes, irritability, changes in sleep or eating habits, fatigue, and an inability to handle daily stress. Other warning signs may surface, such as avoiding friends and social activities that one used to enjoy and having trouble relating to others. One may experience various physical ailments such as headaches or stomach pains without an obvious physical cause. Heavy use of drugs and alcohol may also indicate a potential mental health problem. In some cases, a person may start having delusions, hallucinations, or thoughts of suicide. People who notice these warning signs in themselves or others should reach out for help.

symptoms may withdraw from family and friends and increasingly isolate themselves, weakening social relationships further.

Dr. Susan Noonan is a certified mental health peer specialist and a long-term depression patient. She has witnessed the stress and strains that a family may feel when one person has a mental illness. She says:

> Dealing with a family member who has a mood disorder or anxiety can require a lot of effort from a family member—at times, it can even be exhausting. It can necessitate anything from dealing with the daily distortions in thinking and behavior, to frequent medical appointments, to added time and expenses devoted to the individual. It can be disruptive to the flow of the entire family's routines and patterns, which is stressful over time. It may entail late night phone

the following semester, the university suspended her for a year. She was devastated.

Srivastava realized she needed help and reached out to Boston University's Center for Psychiatric Rehabilitation. She met Courtney Joly-Lowdermilk, a college coach and manager of NITEO, a semester-long program that teaches students resilience, wellness, and academic skills. The NITEO program coaches students countrywide who are on leave from their schools for mental health reasons. Srivastava enrolled in NITEO, where she was able to talk about her mental health and learn strategies to help her cope with the stress and anxiety she had been feeling. "Courtney checks with me when I have depressive bouts," she says. "I definitely still feel like I did sometimes, but things have improved a lot—antidepressants have helped—but being able to talk about it was the most healing aspect. Not doing well was something I thought I would die with."[17] With the skills to manage her mental health, Srivastava plans to return to Boston University full time.

Strain on Relationships

Mental illnesses like depression or anxiety can also significantly strain relationships with family and friends. When a person has a mental illness, it often has a ripple effect on his or her family, creating stress, tension, uncertainty, and a range of emotions from guilt to anger.

Many mental health conditions first surface when people are in their teens or early twenties. Often, many of those individuals still live with their families when their mental health symptoms emerge. As a result, family members and close friends may take on caring for a person struggling with mental health concerns. Most of the time, they do so with little training or support, which can lead to stress. Differences in understanding mental illness and how to treat it can lead to disagreements, anger, and family strain. Even if a person no longer lives in the family home, his or her mental health symptoms can still strain relationships with family and friends. To avoid conflict, people dealing with mental health that would have helped her return to the job. "I think more understanding of the illness would have helped him to understand that I couldn't just put a date on recovery and would have then also eased the pressure I felt to return as quickly as possible,"[14] she says.

Difficulty in School

For young people still in school, mental illness can cause serious disruption and difficulty in their studies. Varsha Srivastava, a twenty-year-old college student, has experienced firsthand the havoc mental illness can cause for students. A high-performing student in high school, Srivastava struggled in her first year at Boston University. She was not happy at the school, and her grades were lower than she wanted, which triggered intense anxiety.

The pressure she put on herself to do well and the increasing anxiety it caused became a vicious cycle. She says:

> The second semester, I said I'd get myself together, but it just got worse. I was so anxious about my grades. Because I was used to being a high-performing student, I couldn't take small steps. I needed to jump in, and I needed to get an A. Every assignment and every class became a huge project that would stress me out so much that I would avoid it because I didn't know how to cope with it.[15]

In her sophomore year, Srivastava's anxiety continued to impact her school performance. "I had no self-confidence, and I had no way to advocate for myself because I was so ashamed of everything," she says. "I would enthusiastically sign up for classes and be excited about the content, and then when I started to slip, I felt like I was not worthy. I'm personable and get along, then I'd hit a bump, and I would see my professors' disappointment and confusion."[16] Her grades plummeted, and the school put her on academic probation. When Srivastava's grades did not improve an update on when she would be able to return to work. "I didn't have an answer; I was unwell and getting more unwell as time was progressing,"[12] she says.

Jayne felt rising pressure to return to work, which increased her anxiety. She stopped answering calls from her employer. Eventually, Jayne's employer sent her a letter asking her to call him with a date for her return to work. Overwhelmed, Jayne called work but told her employer that she could not give him a return date. "I said that I couldn't give him a date because I didn't know and so I wouldn't return at all," she says. "Officially, it sounds as though I resigned, but it didn't feel that way at the time, it felt as though I was cornered to make a decision, one I didn't feel equipped nor well enough to make."[13]

Today Jayne admits that she should have told her employer about her mental health diagnosis. Had she done so, Jayne believes that her employer may have made some accommodations

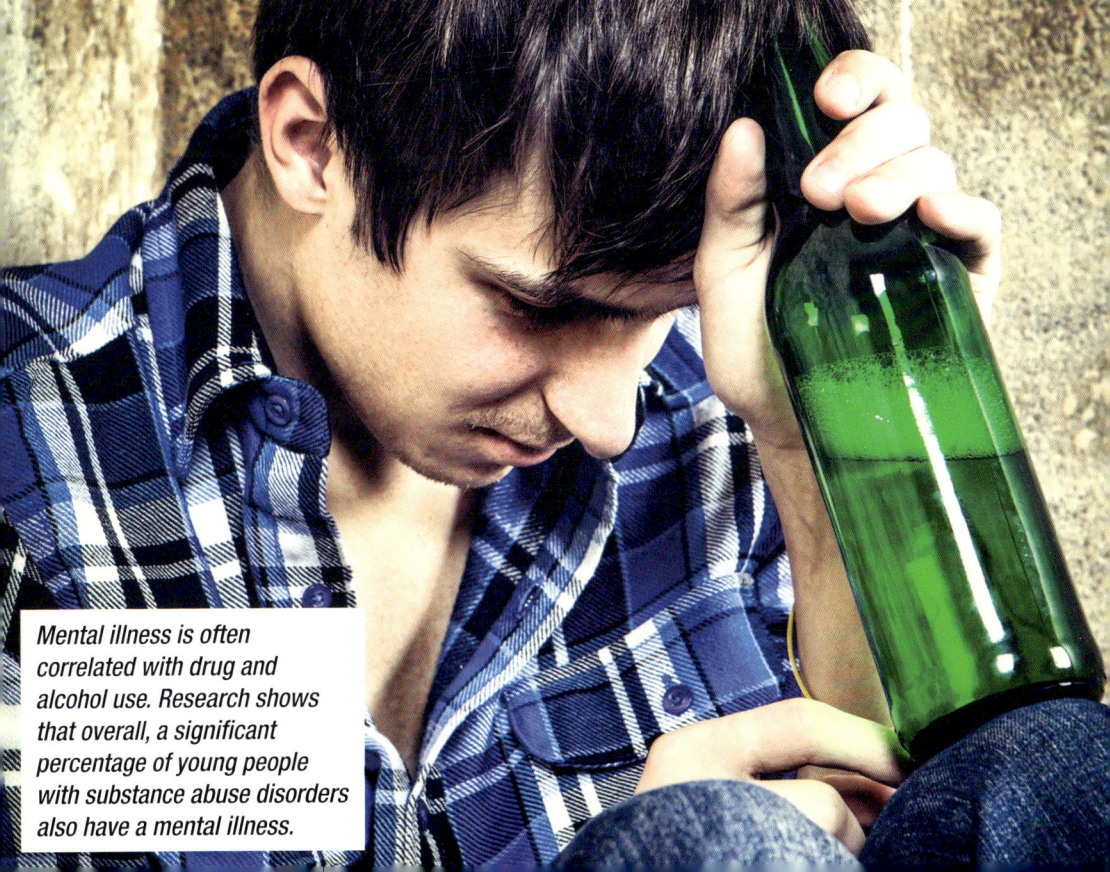

Mental illness is often correlated with drug and alcohol use. Research shows that overall, a significant percentage of young people with substance abuse disorders also have a mental illness.

At the time, I was working as an accounts assistant, preparing accounts and payroll. I was struggling to make it into work (it was an hour's commute), and on the days that it felt impossible, I would call in sick but say it was because of a physical illness. This was happening more and more frequently. I was definitely distracted at work and less productive than I had been, which mattered as we would have to work to time budgets on jobs.[11]

Because Jayne felt ashamed of her depression diagnosis, she tried to hide it from people at work. She never told her employer or manager about her mental health struggles. Instead, she explained her absences with vague sick notes from her doctor. As her absences mounted, Jayne's employer phoned her to ask for

Electroconvulsive Therapy

Electroconvulsive therapy (ECT) is a treatment that can be used for several types of mental illness, including severe depression and severe mania. In an ECT procedure, doctors place the patient under general anesthesia and pass small electric currents through the patient's brain, which triggers a short seizure. ECT can be successful when other mental health treatments have failed because it appears to prompt changes in brain chemistry, which can quickly relieve certain symptoms of mental health disorders. There is some stigma linked to ECT because early attempts to use the treatment administered high doses of electricity without anesthesia. Patients experienced memory loss, fractured bones, and other significant side effects. Today, however, doctors administer ECT in a controlled setting that minimizes risks and makes the procedure much safer. While ECT can be a life-changing treatment for some people, it may not work for everyone.

Mental illness is a leading cause of disability worldwide. Untreated, it can cause problems in a person's daily life. It can disrupt school or work and strain relationships with family and friends. Mental illness also affects people physically. For example, people with depression have a 40 percent increased risk of developing cardiovascular and metabolic diseases compared to people without depression. For those dealing with serious mental illnesses, the risk of these diseases increases to nearly twice that of the general population.

Mental illness can also lead to drug and alcohol use, making a person more likely to develop a substance use disorder. In 2020 nearly one-third (32.1 percent) of American adults with mental illness also had a substance use disorder, according to the NAMI. The connection may be stronger for youth, and research suggests that many adolescents with substance use disorders also have a mental illness. According to the National Institute on Drug Abuse, more than 60 percent of adolescents in substance use disorder treatment programs meet criteria for another mental illness.

Career and Financial Instability

Without treatment, mental illness can disrupt a person's daily life and impact the ability to hold a job successfully. When mental illness prevents working, people can lose income and other job benefits such as health insurance and retirement savings plans. Over time, this can lead to financial instability and poverty. In some cases the lack of a job and steady income can result in homelessness.

Jayne, a thirty-five-year-old accounting assistant in the United Kingdom, knows firsthand how mental illness can derail a career. When she was twenty-two years old, Jayne was diagnosed with depression. At the time, she had been struggling with her mental health but believed she was experiencing a sad mood that would pass eventually. Before long, however, Jayne's depression began to affect her performance at work. She says:

I know that this illness may be with me for a long time,"[9] she says. To cope and manage her mental health, she meets with her therapist regularly, takes medication, exercises, and meditates. She also speaks out to help others better understand depression and give those living with depression hope for recovery. She still has ups and downs, but she knows that she will feel better again with hard work and treatment. "The good news is that I recovered and expect to recover again,"[10] she says.

Mental Health Disorders

Many people feel sad, are anxious, or have other mental health concerns from time to time. However, normal sadness or anxiety can become a problem when symptoms affect the ability to function in daily life. When this occurs, a person may have a mental health disorder.

There are more than two hundred types of mental health disorders. Among the most common, according to the National Alliance on Mental Illness (NAMI): 19.1 percent of American adults have an anxiety disorder; 8.4 percent suffer from depression; 3.6 percent have post-traumatic stress disorder, and 2.8 percent have bipolar disorder.),

Mental health experts believe that mental health disorders are caused by a complex combination of biological, genetic, and environmental factors. For each person, the causes of mental illness are unique. One person's depression may be due to changes in brain chemicals, while another person's depression may be triggered by a traumatic event in his or her life.

A Leading Cause of Disability

Mental illness affects millions of Americans every year. In 2020 nearly 53 million people, about one in five American adults, experienced some form of mental illness, according to the NAMI. Also, one in six American youth ages six to seventeen experience a mental health disorder each year.

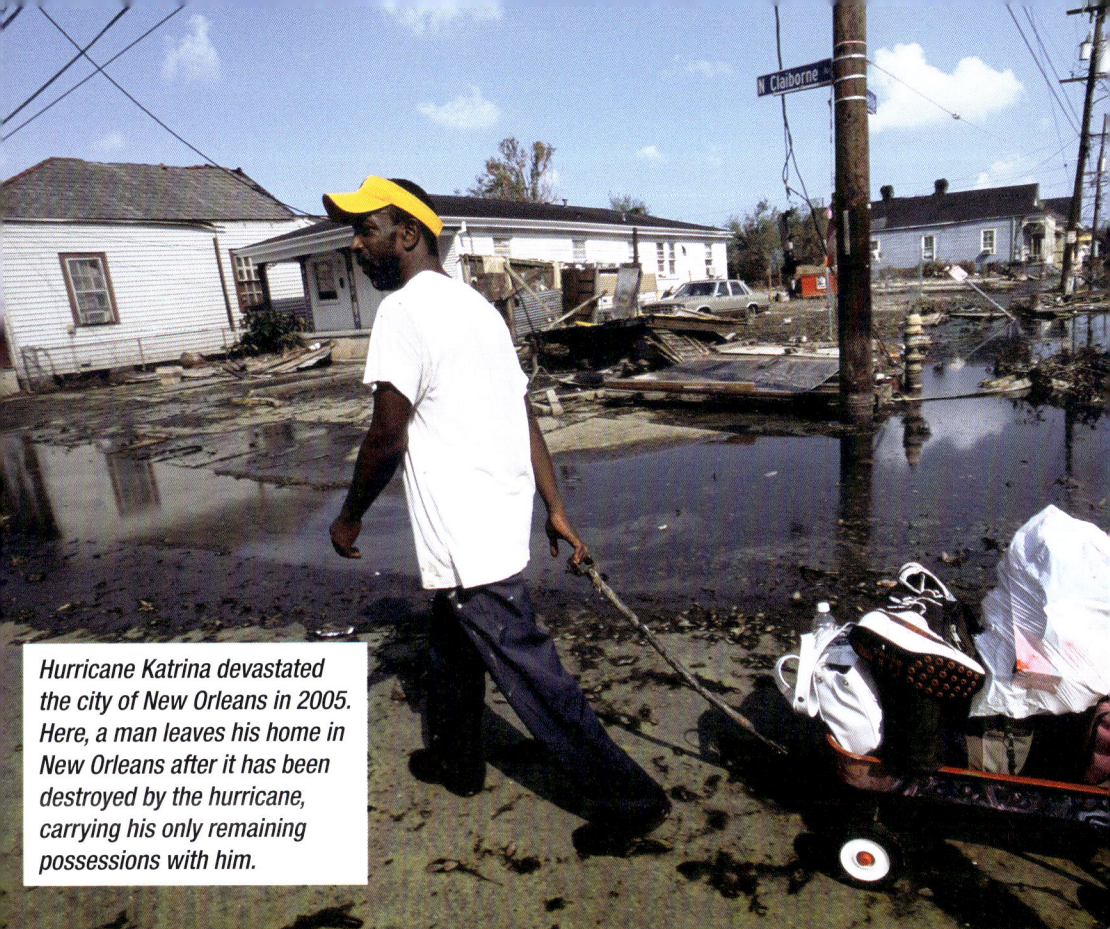

Hurricane Katrina devastated the city of New Orleans in 2005. Here, a man leaves his home in New Orleans after it has been destroyed by the hurricane, carrying his only remaining possessions with him.

group therapy. Over the course of six months, Super was hospitalized five times, yet she still struggled. She tried electroconvulsive therapy—in which a current is passed through the brain while the patient is anesthetized—based on a friend's recommendation. "I was reluctant. However, as I had been unable to work for more than six months and knew that my family was deeply worried about me, I decided to give it a try. It ended up saving my life," she says. "It was as if my brain was jump-started. It made me feel better almost immediately, and I felt nearly recovered by the fourth treatment."[8]

At first, Super thought that she had conquered her depression. Years went by without any significant problems. But then in 2016, while working long, stressful hours, she began to spiral again, and her depression symptoms returned in force. Super learned that depression often returns, with 50 percent of those who recover from a first episode having additional episodes in their lifetime. "So

CHAPTER ONE

A View into Mental Illness

For nearly twenty years, Washington, DC, resident Nora Super has struggled with depression. Her first episode occurred in 2005, when she was a single mom struggling to go to school, work full time, and raise two young children. She had trouble sleeping and felt increasingly sad and anxious. Then Hurricane Katrina devastated her hometown of New Orleans, where many friends and relatives still lived. The images of Katrina's devastation caused Super to sink into depression. "I couldn't think straight. My thoughts went round and round in a spiral. I had less and less energy and was unable to concentrate on my work. Eventually, I couldn't get out of bed in the morning, and it took a tremendous amount of energy just to take a shower,"[7] she says. It got so bad that Super became convinced that her family would be better off if she committed suicide.

Super sought help from mental health professionals. She saw a therapist and psychiatrist regularly and tried various antidepressant medications. She attended cognitive behavioral

> "I couldn't think straight. My thoughts went round and round in a spiral. I had less and less energy and was unable to concentrate on my work. Eventually, I couldn't get out of bed in the morning, and it took a tremendous amount of energy just to take a shower."[7]
>
> —Nora Super, a woman with depression

Getting Help for Mental Illness

Mental health impacts every part of life and is essential to overall health. While mental illness is a serious and growing problem, there is hope. Most people diagnosed with a mental health condition can get better. With treatment, most find relief from their symptoms and live a gratifying life. Treatment may include psychotherapy, medication, and support groups. Often the most effective treatment plans are customized for individual needs. Nutrition, exercise, and activities such as creative arts may also play a role in improving mental health. It is important to remember that treatment and recovery take time. And for most, the first step is getting help.

understand mental health challenges reach into every American family,"[5] said New York City mayor Bill de Blasio in 2020.

Mental Health and Youth

Young adults and their mental health have been hit particularly hard during the coronavirus pandemic. In the same Kaiser Family Foundation survey, more than half (56 percent) of young adults ages eighteen to twenty-four reported anxiety or depression symptoms during the pandemic. Many young adults struggled with mental health as they navigated measures implemented to slow the spread of the coronavirus, including the closures of schools, universities, businesses, and recreational facilities. Suddenly, these young people faced job and income loss and social isolation, and their mental health suffered.

In December 2021 the US surgeon general, Dr. Vivek Murthy, issued an advisory about the mental health crisis affecting the country's youth. Before the coronavirus pandemic, mental health challenges were the leading cause of disability and poor life outcomes in youth, with as many as one in five young people ages three to seventeen having a mental, emotional, developmental, or behavioral disorder. The pandemic added further stress and strain to the mental health of America's youth. Said Murthy in December 2021:

> Mental health challenges in children, adolescents, and young adults are real and widespread. Even before the pandemic, an alarming number of young people struggled with feelings of helplessness, depression, and thoughts of suicide—and rates have increased over the past decade. The COVID-19 pandemic further altered their experiences at home, school, and in the community, and the effect on their mental health has been devastating. The future well-being of our country depends on how we support and invest in the next generation.[6]

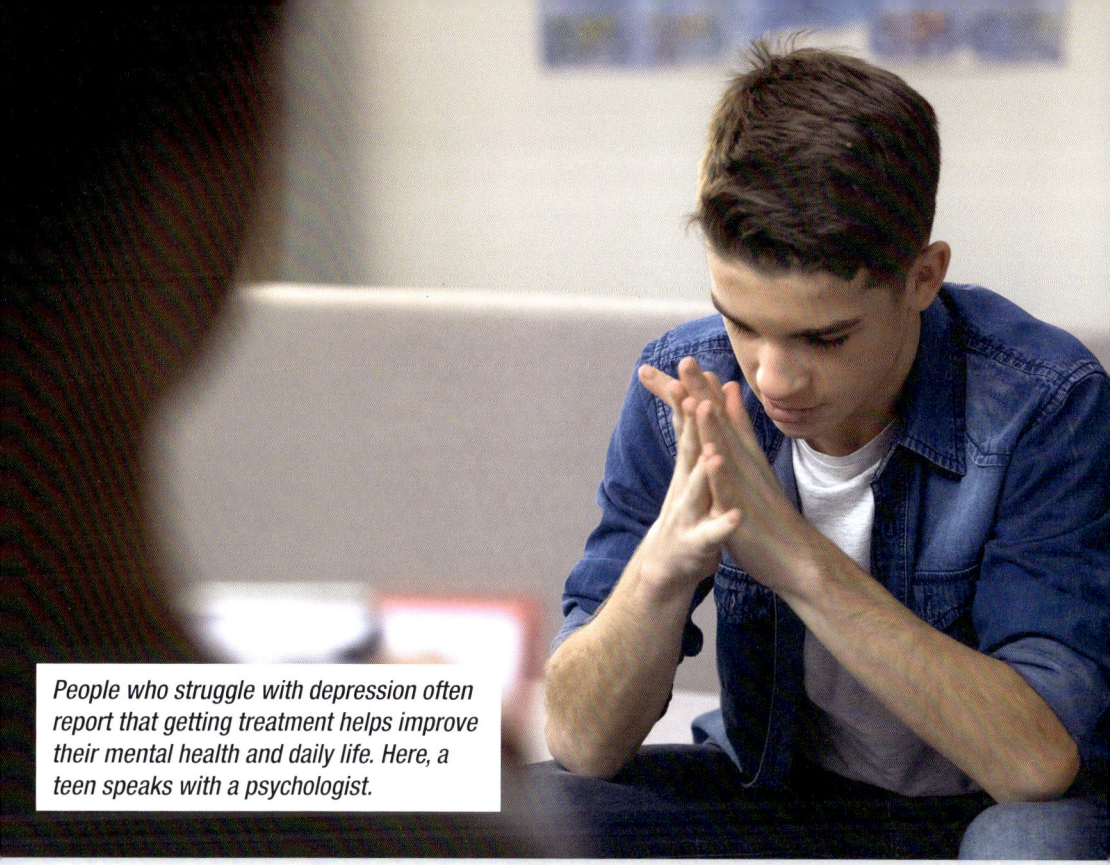

People who struggle with depression often report that getting treatment helps improve their mental health and daily life. Here, a teen speaks with a psychologist.

extreme and volatile mood swings. They might feel more sad or anxious than usual. For others, mental illness can cause problems thinking, communicating with others, or having strange thoughts and feelings.

Mental health disorders are common across the country. In any given year, an estimated 44 million Americans suffer from some form of mental illness, according to Mental Health America. Those numbers have only increased during the coronavirus pandemic, which arrived in the United States in early 2020. According to a poll by the Kaiser Family Foundation, approximately four in ten adults in the United States reported anxiety or depression symptoms in January 2021, compared to one in ten adults who reported the same symptoms during January to June 2019. "I think during the coronavirus, people have come to

> "People have come to understand mental health challenges reach into every American family."[5]
>
> —Bill de Blasio, former New York City mayor

While on temporary leave from school, Harry started cognitive behavioral therapy (CBT) to treat his depression. CBT is a type of talk therapy, or psychotherapy, a common treatment for depression. CBT is based on the idea that people's thoughts influence their feelings and behaviors, and negative thoughts will lead to negative feelings and behaviors. Therefore, CBT attempts to change a person's pattern of negative thinking and behaviors.

> "Accepting that I needed help and that I was unable to continue my studies at that point was an unbelievably difficult decision, but taking a break to focus on my mental health, to recover, has been so much better for me in the long run."[2]
>
> —Harry, a student who lives with depression

For Harry, finally seeking treatment for his depression was the best decision. "CBT helped me understand what was causing my depression and that withdrawing from society and wallowing in self-pity was only making me feel worse. Changing my attitude and adopting a positive outlook for the future, seeing myself in a position where I understood my depression and where it did not have an uncontrollable impact on my day-to-day life, was life-changing,"[3] he says.

Slowly, Harry was able to rebuild his routine and daily life. He started a part-time job at the Mental Health Foundation, a United Kingdom–based charity that strives to help people understand, protect, and sustain mental health. Since starting depression treatment, Harry has seen a significant improvement in his mental health and daily life. "Dealing with depression is an everyday struggle. It's definitely true that some days are worse than others, but I've learned to manage it, to become aware of my symptoms, my triggers, and to remain in control,"[4] he says.

Mental Illness: A Growing Problem

Mental illnesses like Harry's depression are brain-based conditions that affect emotions, thinking, and behavior. For some people, mental illness changes their brain, so they experience

INTRODUCTION

An Everyday Struggle

Depression has long been an everyday struggle for Harry, a British student. When Harry started his university studies, his depression worsened. "When my depression reached its peak, I would progressively miss more and more lectures and seminars, leave social outings early or skip them altogether, spend more and more time alone in self-imposed isolation, and tell myself that it was just because I'm introverted, or that I was 'tired.' And I was tired, but not for lack of sleep; this was actually a symptom of my depression,"[1] says Harry.

Although he had been seeing a doctor for several years, Harry had always refused mental health treatment, thinking he did not need it. Yet by April 2017 Harry's depression had overwhelmed him. He spent days lying in bed, barely eating or drinking, and refusing to socialize with friends. Unable to manage daily life, he considered a temporary withdrawal from school.

At this low point in his life, Harry finally accepted that he needed help for his depression, and it became the first big step toward getting better. "Accepting that I needed help and that I was unable to continue my studies at that point was an unbelievably difficult decision, but taking a break to focus on my mental health, to recover, has been so much better for me in the long run,"[2] he says.

CONTENTS

Introduction — 4
An Everyday Struggle

Chapter One — 9
A View into Mental Illness

Chapter Two — 21
Overcoming the Stigma of Mental Illness

Chapter Three — 32
Getting Treatment

Chapter Four — 44
Lifelong Strategies

Source Notes	55
Getting Help and Information	58
For Further Research	60
Index	61
Picture Credits	64
About the Author	64

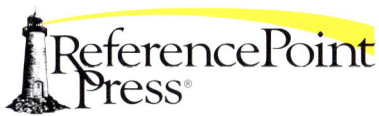

© 2023 ReferencePoint Press, Inc.
Printed in the United States

For more information, contact:
ReferencePoint Press, Inc.
PO Box 27779
San Diego, CA 92198
www.ReferencePointPress.com

ALL RIGHTS RESERVED.
No part of this work covered by the copyright hereon may be reproduced or used in any form or by any means—graphic, electronic, or mechanical, including photocopying, recording, taping, web distribution, or information storage retrieval systems—without the written permission of the publisher.

LIBRARY OF CONGRESS CATALOGING-IN-PUBLICATION DATA

Names: Mooney, Carla, 1970- author.
Title: Getting help : coping with and overcoming mental illness / by Carla
  Mooney.
Description: San Diego, CA : ReferencePoint Press, 2023. | Includes
  bibliographical references and index.
Identifiers: LCCN 2022003808 (print) | LCCN 2022003809 (ebook) | ISBN
  9781678203382 (library binding) | ISBN 9781678203399 (ebook)
Subjects: LCSH: Mental illness. | Mental illness--Treatment.
Classification: LCC RC454 .M664 2023 (print) | LCC RC454 (ebook) | DDC
  616.89--dc23/eng/20220203
LC record available at https://lccn.loc.gov/2022003808
LC ebook record available at https://lccn.loc.gov/2022003809

GETTING HELP
Coping with and Overcoming Mental Illness

Carla Mooney

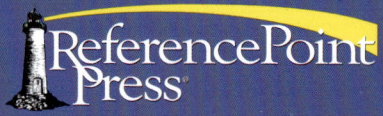

San Diego, CA